Manual
of
Medical Nutrition Therapy

A Nutrition Guide for Long Term Care in Louisiana

7th edition

Edited by:
Brigett L. Scott, PhD, RDN, LDN

Louisiana Dietetic Association
Manual of Medical Nutrition Therapy

A Nutrition Guide for Long Term Care in Louisiana

Compiled by:

The Louisiana Academy of Nutrition and Dietetics Medical Nutrition Therapy
Manual Committees

First Edition, 1984
Deon Gines, PhD, LDN, RD, Chairman; Susan Christian, MS, LDN, RD; Jane Conley, MPH, LDN, RD; Phyllis McCown, MS, LDN; Emma Kate Stiles, MS, RD; Nancy Tolman, PhD, LDN, RD; Ellouise Way, MS, LDN, RD

Second Edition, 1990
Nancy Tolman, PhD, LDN, RD 1987-88 Chairman; Lisa Stansbury, LDN, RD, 1988-89 Chairman; Clare Miller, MS, LDN, RD, 1989-1900 Chairman; Eleanor Ballard, MS, LDN, RD; Anna Barton, LDN, RD; Lana Benson, LDN, RD; Karen Brewton, MA, LDN, RD; Jane Conley, MPH, LDN, RD; Avid Domingue, MA, LDN, RD; Yvette Rothaermel, LDN, RD; Rosemary Schoelen, LDN, RD

Third Edition, 1995
Kathlene A. Lovretich, MMSc, LDN, RD Chairman Peggy Arcement, MS, LDN, RD; Karen Brewton, MA, LDN, RD; Joan Chastain, CDE, LDN, RD; Pam Dalton, CDE, LDN, RD; Diane Douglas, LDN, RD; Lydia Feigler, LDN, RD; Leslie Fontenot, LDN, RD; Jacqueline Gamble, MPH, LDN, RD; Linda Greco, LDN, RD; Brenda Janes, CDM; Mary Ann Kaylor, MMSc, LDN, RD, CNSD LDN, RD; Mary Beth O'Donnell, MS, MBA; Marsha Piacun, MBA, LDN, RD; Elaine Rowzee, LDN, RD; Suzette Sanders, LDN, RD

Fourth Edition, 2001 – Renamed LDA Manual of Medical Nutrition Therapy
Beth Fontenot, MS, LDN, RD 2001 Chairman; Marie LeBlanc, LDN, RD 1999-2001 Chairman; Amy Yates, LDN, RD 1998-1999 Chairman; Lydia Hampton, LDN, RD 1997 Chairman; Mary Ann Kaylor, MMSc, LDN, RD, CNSD 1996 Chairman; Kimberly Faulk, LDN, RD Jacqueline Gamble, MPH, LDN, RD; Monica Gauthier, Med, RD, CNSD; Linda Greco, LDN, RD; Paula Rhodes, LDN, RD; Lynn Schumacher, MPH, RD, LDN; Lea Theriot, MS, LDN, RD

Fifth Edition, 2005
Beth Fontenot, MS, LDN, RD, Chairman; Mandy Armentor, LDN, RD; Ginger Bouvier, MEd, LDN, RD; Sara Butler, LDN, RD; Valerie Calhoun, MS, LDN, RD; Jessica Coffee, LDN, RD; Judy Dupuis, RD; Jo Jo Dantone-DeBarbieris, MS, LDN RD, CDE; Kim Fowler, MS, LDN, RD; Linda Massey, RD; Deborah Oglesby, LDN, RD; Martha Palotta, LDN, RD, CDE; Rebecca Richardson, LDN, RD; Morgan Roberie, LDN, RD; Sandy Sutton- Broussard, LDN, RD; Lea Theriot, MS, LDN, RD; Rita Walker, MS, LDN, RD; Paula Weeks, MS, LDN, RD

Sixth Edition, 2010

Carol E. O'Neil, PhD, MPH, LDN, RD, Chairman and Prithiva Chanmugam, PhD, LDN, RD. This project also included a service-learning project with the 2008-2009 Louisiana State University School of Human Ecology Medical Nutrition Therapy Students: Julie Aldridge, Sabrina Bauggue, Brooke Bayham, Stratton Beatrous, Leah Beauchamp, Amilyn Bonnette, Camille Broome, Emily Brown, Tap Bui, Leslie Cenac, Alexandra Cobb, Megan Deal, Adele Dorgant, Heather Duby, Allison Erdly, Kayla Frey, Leslie Freyer, Holly Gaines, Sandlin Goebel, Anna Graml, Mary Gray, Casey Guillory, Lauren Hayes, Christine Henson, Melissa Henderson, Dylandra Holden, Caroline Holland, Mary Holland, Darryl Holliday, Kelly Hughes, Angela Jurma, Brittany Kingsley, Kelli Lee, Jennifer Lew, M. Marion Marsh, Jamie Mascari, Joseph McLean, Cali Meyer, Julie Miller, Danielle Millet, Christiana Moore, Elizabeth Nordman, Laura Petitt, Candida Rebello, Alayna Rockenschuh, Emily Routh, Stephanie Smith, Megan Thibodeaux, Allison Tipler, M. Elise Torres, Aneesha Virani, Jessica West, Ashley Williams, and Elizabeth Worthey.

In addition, the following individuals worked on this edition: Jo Ann Puls, MS, LDN, RD, Brandi Milioto, MS, LDN, RD, Cathy Vinci, MS, RD, Hollie Eskew, MS, RD, Jamie Bissett, LDN, RD, and Michael Zanovec, MS, and Hollie Barr.

Seventh Edition, 2015

Brigett L. Scott, PhD RDN LDN, Chairman, Elizabeth Sloan, MS RDN, LDN, Sherry Foret, MS, RDN, LDN, and Tammy Bourque, MS RDN, LDN.

ISBN-13: 978-1515392422

ISBN-10: 1515392422

ACKNOWLEDGMENTS

The *Louisiana Dietetic Association Diet Manual*, 1984 edition, was completed under the supervision of the LDA Diet Manual Committee. The manual was field tested by consultant dietitians in the state.

Deon Gines, PhD, LDN, RD, and Nancy Tolman, PhD, LDN, RD, College of Human Ecology, Louisiana Tech University, served as advisors during the planning, testing, and preparation of the 1984 manual.

The 1990 edition of the manual was completed with the assistance of three teams of LDA Diet Manual Committees. In addition to thanking all the members of the Diet Manual Committees, thanks are also extended to the following people who contributed to the revision of the manual:

Zoe Crumpler, LDN, RD; Ruth Gaspard, LDN, RD; Charles Feutch, PD, FACP; Ruby George, CDM; Melissa Hill, LDN, RD; Alice Landry, LDN, RD; Joan S. LeBouef, LDN, RD; Karen Perkins, LDN, RD; Marsha E. Piacun, LDN, RD; Joy Regan, LDN, RD; Eunice Ritchie, MS, RPh; Louise Schewe, MS, LDN, RD; Carmel Veron, LDN, RD; and Ruby Watts, CDM

The 1995 edition could not have happened without the dedication, expertise, time and talent of all the section writers:

Peggy Arcement, MS, LDN, RD; Karen Brewton, MA, LDN, RD; Joan Chastain, CDE, LDN, RD; Pam Dalton, LDN, RD, CDE; Diane Douglas, LDN, RD; Lydia Feigler, LDN, RD; Leslie Fontenot, LDN, RD; Jacqueline Gamble, MPH, LDN, RD; Linda Greco, LDN, RD; Brenda James, CDM; Mary Ann Kaylor, MMSc, LDN, RD, CNSD; Mary Beth O'Donnell, MS, MBA,LDN, RD; Elaine Rowzee, LDN, RD; and Suzette Sanders, LDN, RD

The *LDA Manual of Medical Nutrition Therapy*, 2001 edition, was the combined effort of many people. In addition to those who worked on revising the sections, (see Table of Contents), the editor would like to thank those who helped with proofreading:

Debra Hollingsworth, PhD, LDN, RD, RS; Mary Trahan, LDN, RD; Pat White, LDN, RD

The 2005 edition was made possible by the following dietitians who volunteered their time and expertise to review and revise the sections.

Beth Fontenot, MS, LDN, RD, Chairman; Mandy Armentor, LDN, RD; Ginger Bouvier, M.Ed, LDN, RD; Sara Butler, LDN, RD; Valerie Calhoun, MS, LDN, RD; Jessica Coffee, LDN, RD; Jo Jo Dantone-DeBarbieris, MS, LDN RD, CDE; Judy Dupuis, RD; Kim Fowler, MS, LDN, RD; Linda Massey, RD; Deborah Oglesby, LDN, RD; Martha Palotta, LDN, RD, CDE; Rebecca Richardson, LDN, RD; Morgan Roberie, LDN, RD; Sandy Sutton-Broussard, LDN, RD Lea Theriot, MS, LDN, RD; Rita Walker, MS, LDN, RD; and Paula Weeks, MS, LDN, RD

The 2010 edition was made possible by:

Carol E. O'Neil, PhD, MPH, LDN, RD; and Prithiva Chanmugam, PhD, LDN, RD, from the faculty of Louisiana State University. Michael Zanovec, MS provided technical assistance. The students in the 2008-2009 Louisiana State University School of Human Ecology Medical Nutrition Therapy service-learning classes provided additional information.

The 2015 edition was made possible by the following dietitians who who volunteered their time and expertise to review and revise the sections.
Brigett Scott, PhD, RDN, LDN; Elizabeth Sloan, MS, RDN, LDN; Sherry Foret, MS, RDN, LDN; and Tammy Borque, MS, RDN, LDN

PREFACE

The 1984 edition of this manual was written primarily for use in small hospitals, nursing homes, and health care facilities throughout Louisiana. The 1990 edition was developed specifically for the long-term care facility. The 1995 edition had the added focus of home health as the home had also become a long-term care setting. The 2001 edition included information on liberalized diets for geriatric patients, a new chapter on nutrition for children with special health care needs, and six patient education handouts. The 2005 edition has a new section on the Gluten Free Diet. The 2010 edition was compiled with a heavy emphasis on the peer-reviewed literature, and, wherever possible, used an evidence based approach. Many of the diseases or conditions did not have an extensive literature so that a purely evidence based approach could not be used. The 2015 version of the manual provides readers with the option of a hard copy or an electronic ebook.

Sections pertaining to the various diets are designed to be used by the Certified Dietary Manager in the facility. Dietary modifications are simplified so that the dietary manager can concentrate on serving nutritious, safe, attractive, tasty meals in a pleasant environment. The section entitled "Nutrition Support" is included to assist the facility's nutritional multi-disciplinary team in identifying patients at nutritional risk and in developing a comprehensive care plan for those residents.

The diet analyses were done using the USDA Database. A single representative menu is presented and may not represent usual intakes. Several diets, including clear liquid, full liquid, and high energy/high protein are intended for short use only. The majority of vitamin A in these diet analyses is from β-carotene. It is important in menu planning to provide a variety of foods to help individuals meet current dietary recommendations.

Table of Contents

Manual of Medical Nutrition Therapy

Approved by:

Institution: _____

Physician, Chief of Staff	Date

Physician	Date

Physician	Date

Licensed Dietitian	Date

Dietary Manager	Date

Administrator	Date

Director of Nursing	Date

NUTRITION ASSESSMENT in Long-Term Care Facilities

Nutritional care of the individual during **long-term care** must be directed toward meeting the mental, social, and physical needs over an extended period of time. These needs change depending upon the emotional and mental status of the individual at the time of the assessment. Identifying the individual who is at possible nutritional risk is an important role of the nutritional assessment. The Joint Commission has a number of requirements related to cultural competence long term care. It is strongly recommended that licensed dietitian/nutritionists review these requirements prior to using this manual. Moreover, a current therapeutic diet manual approved by the dietitian and medical staff must be readily available to all medical, nursing, and food service staff. For disease specific care, a dietitian is needed.

TIME FRAME

All residents residing in a long-term care facility are required to have a nutritional assessment completed within 14 days of admission.
1. At least annually thereafter, nutritional assessments must be completed on all residents.
2. Following any change in the resident's status, a new nutritional assessment must be completed.

NUTRITION SCREENING ROLES

Administrator

1. Ensures nutritional assessment and screening systems are in place.
2. Ensures adequacy of staff to implement and maintain system.

Physician

1. Writes diet orders.
2. Assumes legal responsibilities for nutritional status of resident.
3. Orders nutrition-related treatments.

Nursing Staff

1. Assists in setting up screening system.
2. Maintains or assists in screening system.
3. Ensures resident consumes food and promotes resident consumption of meal plan.
4. Organizes and distributes workload.
5. Determines timing of feeder trays.
6. Determines appropriate timing of staff breaks as they relate to the nutrition care plan.
7. Records accurate and meaningful information about resident's food and fluid intake.

Dietary Manager

1. Ensures:
   a. Food is safe and nutritious.
   b. Food is palatable and attractive.
   c. Diets are served accurately.
   d. Substitutions are appropriate.
2. Screens each resident.
3. Interviews residents and family members, as appropriate, regarding food preferences.
4. Monitors food and fluid intake and plate waste.
5. Alerts licensed dietitian/nutritionist, physician, nurse, and others to problems noted.

Licensed **Dietitian**/Nutritionist

1. Reviews resident screens.
2. Monitors system.
3. Performs nutrition assessments.
4. Records findings, recommendations, and follow-up comments in medical record.
5. Alerts multi-disciplinary team members of nutrition-related problems.
6. Assists in implementing screening system; trains personnel on use of these systems.

Table 1-1. Responsibilities of a Dietary Manager and a Licensed Dietitian/Nutritionist in Long-term care facilities.	
Dietary Manager	**Licensed Dietitian/Nutritionist**
Nutritional Screening Data Collection	
1. Completes consultant dietitian referral form based on nutritional risk list. 2. Completes screening.	1. Reviews referral form. Collects additional data from dietary manager, nursing service, and others to determine progress and problems since last visit for assessment. 2. Reviews screening.
Nutritional Assessment Data Collection	
	3. Completes nutrition assessment and certifies the accuracy and completeness.
Documentation of Data	
3. Screening should be done at least quarterly.	4. Frequency varies, at least annually on low-risk residents; however, high-risk patients, such as those on enteral feeds should be assessed at least monthly
Follow-Up	
4. Follow up should be done at least quarterly.	5. Frequency varies: monthly, quarterly, or annually, as needed.

NUTRITION ASSESSMENT in Acute Care Facilities

Nutritional care of the individual during **acute care** must be directed toward meeting the mental, social, and physical needs of patients or clients. These needs change depending upon the emotional and mental status of the individual at the time of the assessment. Identifying the individual who is at possible nutritional risk is an important role of the nutritional assessment.

The Joint Commission requires that nutrition screening be conducted in acute care facilities within 24 hours of admission. Nutrition screening can be conducted by a registered nurse, a dietetic technician registered (DTR) or a licensed dietitian/nutritionist. There is no specific screening program or form. A critical access hospital must have a dietitian full time/part time or on a consultant basis. Moreover, a current therapeutic diet manual approved by the dietitian and medical staff is readily available to all medical, nursing, and food service staff. For disease specific care, a dietitian is needed.

NUTRITIONAL RISK FACTORS

Feeding Related:
Chewing difficulties
Swallowing difficulties--consult speech pathologist for further assessment if patient has dysphagia
Food intake less than 75%
Mechanically-altered diet order
Failure to eat foods from all five food groups
Tube fed
Significant food allergy or food aversions

Weight:
Underweight - 10 to 15% or more below desirable weight
Significant unplanned, undesirable weight loss (see below)
Overweight - 15 to 30% above desirable weight
Edema and/or ascites

Deranged lab values:
Serum albumin or pre-albumin, CRP, blood glucose, HgB A1C, blood urea nitrogen, hematocrit or hemoglobin
Illness:
Frequent nausea or vomiting
Diarrhea/Chronic constipation
Decubitus ulcers
Cancer or cancer therapy
Recent trauma
Infection, burn, fever, or surgery

Hemodialysis
Type 1 diabetes or type 2 diabetes that requires insulin

Debilities:
Inability to communicate
Visually impaired
Dependent feeder

Other:
Age
Polypharmacy
Inability to conduct activities of daily living
Social isolation**PROGRESS NOTE DOCUMENTATION**

Dietary Manager

1. Diet order confirmation.
2. Percentage of intake: Changes and results of food audits completed.
3. Acceptance or rejection of foods: Changes and diet compliance.
4. Weight status: Changes and percent of desirable body weight.
5. Changes in feeding, chewing, and swallowing abilities, in table seating, or at meal time.
6. Diet or nutrition education with resident or family.
7. Snacks, nutritional supplements, or special food items (state item, frequency, time, and percent intake of acceptance)
8. Skin condition, as related to decubitus ulcers.
9. Progress made since last care plan conference.
10. Diabetes status, if relevant.
11. Adaptive feeding equipment (item, training, and acceptance).
12. Recommendations on appropriate diet order, including consistency.

Licensed Dietitian/Nutritionist – utilizing the Nutrition Care Process

1. Weight evaluation.
2. Nutrition-related lab value assessment.
3. Nutrient-drug interaction assessment.
4. Nutrition assessment
5. Dietary counseling for resident or family, as appropriate.
6. Accuracy and completeness of food intake and weight records.
7. Calculation, if appropriate, of energy, protein, baseline fluid needs, and tube feeding diet order.
8. Review of nursing and physician notes, if appropriate.
9. Diet order and consistency evaluation.
10. Recommendations on appropriate diet order, consistency, fluid needs, energy needs, supplementation, lab studies, vitamin-mineral supplementation, and weight record.

CALCULATION OF ENERGY, PROTEIN, AND FLUID NEEDS IN ADULTS

Table 1.2 Energy Needs – Estimating Resting Energy [1,2]

Calculation	Male	Female	Units
Mifflin-St. Jeor	RMR = (9.99 X weight) + (6.25 X height) – (4.92 X age) + 5	RMR = (9.99 X weight) + (6.25 X height) – (4.92 X age) – 161	Equations use weight in kilograms and height in centimeters and age in years.
Ireton-Jones 1997 Equation	REE = (5 x weight) – (11 x age) + (244 if male) + (239 if trauma present) + (840 if burns present) + 1784		
Harris-Benedict Equation	BMR = 66.5 + (13.8 x weight) + (5 x height) – (6.8 x age)	BMR = 655.1 + (9.6 x weight) + (1.9 x height) – (4.7 x age)	

To determine total daily energy needs, the RMR must be multiplied by the appropriate activity factor:
- 1.200 = sedentary (little or no exercise)
- 1.375 = lightly active (light exercise/sports 1-3 days/week)
- 1.550 = moderately active (moderate exercise/sports 3-5 days/week)
- 1.725 = very active (hard exercise/sports 6-7 days a week)
- 1.900 = extra active (very hard exercise/sports and physical job)

Then subtract 500 to 1,000 calories to lose 1 to 2 pounds per week. However, total energy needs should seldom be less than 1,200 kcals/day.

Table 1.3 The National Academy of Sciences, Institute of Medicine, and Food and Nutrition Board, in partnership with Health Canada, have developed estimated energy needs for adults. [3]

Estimated energy expenditure (EER) = total energy expenditure (TEE)	
For males 19 years and older (body mass index [BMI] 18.5-25 kg/m^2])	EER = 662 – (9.53 x age [y]) + PA (15.91 x weight [kg] + 539.6 x height [m])
For overweight and obese males 19 years and older (BMI ≥25 kg/m^2)	TEE = 1086 – (10.1 x age [y] + PA x (13.7 x weight [kg] + 416 x height [m]
For normal and overweight or obese males 19	TEE = 864 – (9.72 x age [y]) + PA (14.2 x

years and older (BMI $\geq$18.5 kg/m^2)	weight [kg] + 503 x height [m])

Where PA is the physical activity coefficient:
PA = 1.00 if PAL is estimated to be >1.0 <1.4 (Sedentary)
PA = 1.11 if PAL is estimated to be >1.4 <1.6 (low active)
PA = 1.25 if PAL is estimated to be >1.6 < 1.9 (active)
PA = 1.48 if PAL is estimated to be >1.9 < 2.5 (very active)

Estimated energy expenditure (EER) = total energy expenditure (TEE)

For females 19 years and older (body mass index [BMI] 18.5-25 kg/m^2])	EER = 354 – (6.91 x age [y]) + PA (9.36 x weight [kg] + 726 x height [m])
For overweight and obese females 19 years and older (BMI $\geq$25 kg/m^2)	TEE = 448 – (7.95 x age [y]) + PA (11.4 x weight [kg] + 619 x height [m])
For normal and overweight or obese females 19 years and older (BMI $\geq$18.5 kg/m^2)	TEE = 387– (7.31 x age [y]) + PA (10.9 x weight [kg] + 660.7 x height [m])

Where PA is the physical activity coefficient:
PA = 1.00 if PAL is estimated to be $\geq$1.0 <1.4 (Sedentary)
PA = 1.14 if PAL is estimated to be $\geq$1.4 <1.6 (low active)
PA = 1.27 if PAL is estimated to be $\geq$1.6 < 1.9 (active)
PA = 1.45 if PAL is estimated to be $\geq$1.9 < 2.5 (very active)

Historically, the Harris-Benedict equation has been used to calculate energy needs; however, some studies have found it overestimates energy needs.[4] In other studies, differences were not significantly different from Mifflin-St. Jeor.[5] Recently modifications have been made for use with the critically ill and calculated energy needs corresponded to measured needs more closely.[6] The Mifflin-St. Jeor equation has been validated over a 10 year period and shown to be the most reliable.[7] Older individuals have been under-represented in studies determining appropriate formulas, thus additional studies are clearly warranted.

Protein Needs

The RDA for maintenance of serum proteins and muscle mass in healthy adults is 0.8 gm/kg body weight (BW).

Protein requirements vary in certain disease states:

- Mild Infection, Minor Surgery: 1.0 - 1.2 gm/kg
- Moderate Infection, Major Surgery: 1.2 - 1.8 gm/kg
- Severe Infection, Major Wounds: 1.5 - 2.0 gm/kg
- Kidney Failure, Pre-dialysis: 0.6 - 0.75 gm/kg
- Kidney Failure, Hemodialysis: 1.1 - 1.4 gm/kg dry weight
- Kidney Failure, Peritoneal Dialysis: 1.2-1.3 gm/kg
- Older Adults: 1.0 - 1.1 gm/kg
- Pressure Sores (Increase with Stage of Sore): 1.2 - 1.5 gm/kg
- Pregnancy and Lactation: 1.1 gm/kg

Fluid Needs

Fluid requirements can generally be estimated at 1 ml/Kcal or 30 ml/kg body weight.

Fluid restrictions may be required for patients with kidney failure, congestive heart failure, or volume overload. Fluid is usually limited to 1,000 ml/day, urine output + 500 mL, or specified by the physician. If the patients are fluid restricted, be sure that the patient has enough fluid remaining to take any meds at bedtime.

OVERVIEW OF HEIGHT AND WEIGHT CALCULATIONS

Calculation of BMI

BMI is calculated the same way for both adults and children. The calculation is based on the following formula:[8]

Table 1.4. Formula and Calculation
Formula: weight (kg) / [height (m)^2]   With the metric system, the formula for BMI is weight in kilograms divided by height in meters squared. Since height is commonly measured in centimeters, divide height in centimeters by 100 to obtain height in meters.   Example: Weight = 68 kg, Height = 165 cm (1.65 m)   Calculation: $68 \div (1.65)^2 = 24.98$ Note. lbs $\div$ 2.2 = kg   in. x 0.0254 = m

Interpretation of BMI for adults[8]

For adults 20 years of age and older, BMI is interpreted using standard weight status categories that are the same for all ages and for both men and women. The standard weight status categories associated with BMI ranges are shown in the following table:

Table 1.5. Body Mass Index, Weight Status, and Health Risk		
BMI	**Weight Status**	**Health Risk**
Below 18.5	Underweight	If <16 possible eating disorder or wasting disease
18.5 – 24.9	Normal	Healthy, low risk
25.0 – 29.9	Overweight	Associated with increased risk of disease
30.0 and Above	Obese	Associated with further increased risk of disease

As an example, here are the weight ranges, the corresponding BMI ranges, and the weight status categories for a sample height.

Table 1.6. Weight Range, Body Mass Index, and Weight Status for a Sample Height			
Height	**Weight Range**	**BMI**	**Weight Status**
5' 9"	124 lbs or less	Below 18.5	Underweight
	125 lbs to 168 lbs	18.5 to 24.9	Normal
	169 lbs to 202 lbs	25.0 to 29.9	Overweight
	203 lbs or more	30 or higher	Obese

How reliable is BMI as an indicator of body fatness?

The correlation between the BMI number and body fatness is fairly strong; however the correlation varies by sex, race, and age.

- At the same BMI, women tend to have more body fat than men.

- At the same BMI, older people, on average, tend to have more body fat than younger adults.

- Highly trained athletes may have a high BMI because of increased muscularity rather than increased body fatness.

It is also important to remember that BMI is only one factor related to risk for disease. For assessing someone's likelihood of developing overweight- or obesity-related diseases, the National Heart, Lung, and Blood Institute guidelines recommend looking at two other predictors:

- Waist circumference since abdominal fat is a predictor of risk for obesity-related diseases.
- Other risk factors the individual has for diseases and conditions associated with obesity (*e.g*, high blood pressure or physical inactivity).

- **Calculate BMI on line from the CDC**

- **The BMI Tables**

BMI in the Elderly

One problem with BMI is that the majority of evidence and the majority of studies have been done on younger adults not in the elderly. For individuals over 65 years of age, the desirable BMI is between 24 and 33.[9] More studies are needed in this age group.[10]

Height Estimation for Non-Ambulatory Residents

Not all individuals in long-term care are able to have a standing height measurement taken. A recumbent board can be used or height can be estimated using arm span, knee height, or sitting height.

Adult recumbent:
1. Stand on the right side of the body.
2. Align the body so that the lower extremities, trunk, shoulders, and head are straight
3. Place a mark at the top of the sheet in line with the crown of the head and one at the bottom of the sheet in line with the base of the heels.
4. Measure the length between marks with measuring tape.

Arm Span:
1. Have the client extend their arms straight out to the sides at a 90°-degree angle from the body.
2. Measure the distance from the longest fingertip of one hand to the longest fingertip of the other hand. (This is an estimation of height that may be 1-2% off of actual height).

Knee Height--the most common approach to estimate height is knee height since it correlates with stature.[11-13] It should be noted that stature decreases with age and that this is more prevalent in women than men and there are cultural/racial differences. [12-19] It is also important to use an accurate caliper.[20]

1. Use the left leg for measurements.
2. Bend the left knee and ankle to 90°; a triangle should be used if one is available.
3. Using knee calipers open the caliper and place the fixed part under the heel. Place the sliding blade down against the thigh, approximately 2 inches behind the patella.
4. Measure from the heel to the anterior surface of the thigh, using a cloth measuring tape.
5. Obtain the measurement and, if necessary, convert inch measurements to centimeters by multiplying by 2.54.
6. Use the following formulas to estimate height from knee height:

Ages 19-60 years:

White Male: Ht (cm) = 71.85 + (1.88 x knee height)
Black Male: Ht (cm) = 73.42 + (1.79 x knee height)
White Female: Ht (cm) = 70.25 + (1.87 x knee height) – (0.06 x age)
Black Female: Ht (cm) = 68.10 + (1.86 x knee height) – (0.06 x age)

Age > 60 years:

White Male: 59.01 + (2.08 x knee height)
Black Male: 95.79 + (1.37 x knee height)
White Female: 75 + (1.91 x knee height) – (0.17 x age)
Black Female: 58.72 + (1.96 x knee height)

Determination of Frame Size

Method 1. Height is recorded with shoes. Wrist circumference is measured just distal to the styloid process at the wrist crease on the right arm, using a tape measure. Then use the following formula:

$$r = \frac{Height\ (cm)}{Wrist\ circumference\ (cm)}$$

Frame size can then be determined:

Table 1.7. Frame Size Calculations for Males and Females using Height and Wrist Corcumference	
Males	**Females**
r > 10.4 small	r > 11.0 small
r = 9.6 - 10.4 small	r = 10.1- 11. small
r < 9.6 large	r < 10.1 large

Method 2. The patients' right arm is extended forward perpendicular to the body, with the arm bent so that the elbow joint is measured with a sliding caliper along the axis of the upper arm on

the two prominent bones on either side of the elbow. This is recorded as the elbow breadth. The tables below provide the measurements for a medium frame; higher measurements connote a large frame and smaller ones connote a small frame.

Table 1.8. Frame Size Calculations for Males and Females using Height and Elbow Breadth			
Males		**Females**	
Height in 1" heels	**Elbow Breadth (in)**	**Height in 1" heels**	**Elbow Breadth (in)**
5'2"-5"3"	2 ½ - ⅞	4'10" - 4"11"	2 ¼ - 2 ½
5'4"-5'7"	2 ⅝-2 ⅞	5'0"-5'3"	2 ¼ - 2 ½
5'8" - 5'11"	2 ¼ -3	5'4"-5'7"	2 ⅜ to 2 ⅝
6'0"-6'3"	2 ¾ - 3 ⅛	5'8"-5'11"	2 ⅜ to 2 ⅝
6'4"	2 ⅞ 3 ¼	6'0"	

Adjustments of Desirable Body Weight for Amputations

The percentages listed below are estimates since body proportions vary in individuals. Use of these percentages provides an average adjustment of a desirable body weight for an individual who has an amputation.

Type of Amputation % of Total Body Weight
Foot 1.5%
Below Knee 5.9%
Above Knee 10.1%
Entire Lower Extremity 16.0%
Hand 0.7%
Below Elbow 2.3%
Entire Upper Extremity 5.0%
Trunk without Extremities 50%

Instructions: Use the resident's approximate height prior to the amputation. Using this height calculate the desirable weight for an adult. Next adjust this weight for the resident's type of amputation. Estimated IBW = $\frac{100 - \% \text{ amputation}}{100}$ x IBW for original height

Example: To determine the desirable body weight for a 5'11" male with a below the knee amputation BKA):

Calculate desirable body weight for a 5'11" male = 172 #
Subtract the weight of the amputated limb (5.9%) = 172 x 0.059 = 10.2#
Desirable weight of a 5'11" male with a BKA = 172 - 10.2 =~ 162#

Of particular import when assessing a patient is weight change. The following formulas can be used for a) percent usual body weight and b) percent weight change.

Percent usual body weight: *Percent weight change:*

   Current weight   x100   Usual body weight - present weight x 100
Usual Body Weight   Usual body weight

Table 1.9. Interpretation of Unintentional Weight Loss[21]		
Time Frame	Significant Weight Loss	Severe Weight Loss
1 week	1-2% UBW	>2% UBW
1 month	5% UBW	>5% UBW
3 months	7.5% UBW	>7.5% UBW
6 months	10% UBW	>10% UBW
Adapted from Nelmes, Sucher, Long. Nutrition Therapy and Pathophysiology.Thompson Wadsworth. 2014		

Or: 100-% usual body weight = % change

Table 1.10. Weight Loss Table, 5% and 10% (all figures in pounds)				
Weight	**5% Loss**	**Result**	**10% Loss**	**Result**
90	4.50	85.50	9.0	81.0
95	4.75	90.25	9.5	85.5
100	5.00	95.00	10.0	90.0
105	5.25	99.75	10.5	94.5
110	5.50	104.50	11.0	99.0
115	5.75	109.25	11.5	103.5
120	6.00	114.00	12.0	108.0
125	6.25	118.75	12.5	112.5
130	6.50	123.50	13.0	117.0
135	6.75	128.50	13.5	121.5
140	7.00	133.00	14.0	126.0
145	7.25	137.75	14.5	130.5
150	7.50	142.50	15.0	135.0
155	7.75	147.25	15.5	139.5
160	8.00	152.00	16.0	144.0
165	8.25	156.75	16.5	148.5
170	8.50	161.50	17.0	153.0
175	8.75	166.25	17.5	157.5
180	9.00	171.00	18.0	162.0
185	9.25	175.75	18.5	166.5
190	9.50	180.50	19.0	171.0
195	9.75	185.25	19.5	175.5
200	10.00	190.00	20.0	180.0
205	10.25	194.75	20.5	184.5
210	10.50	199.50	21.0	189.0
215	10.75	204.25	21.5	193.5
220	11.00	209.00	22.0	198.0

SKINFOLD MEASUREMENTS

The most widely used method of estimating indirect percent body fat is to measure skinfolds--or the thickness of a double fold of skin and compressed subcutantous adipose tissue. When done correctly, skinfolds provide estimates of body composition that correlate well with other methods. Triceps skinfolds are taken at the midline on the back of the arm over the triceps muscle between the acromion process of the scapula and the olecranon process of the ulna. Accuracy in defining the exact point is critical.[22-23]

In the US, most skinfolds are taken on the right side of the body; whereas, in Europe, they are taken on the left side. A minimum of two measurements should be taken 15 seconds apart and measurements should be averaged. The triceps skinfolds are commonly obtained in population surveys, such as the National Health and Nutrition Examination Survey; other skinfold include the subsapular, midmaxillary, the suprailiac, the abdomen, the thigh, and the medial calf. Recumbent measurements can be taken while the patient is lying on either side. Most nutrition assessment textbooks explain the procedures for taking these measurements.

Midarm Circumference

Midarm circumference can be used in equations to calculate arm muscle area an estimated body weight.[24-26] Midarm circumference is the circumference of the upper arm at the site the triceps skin fold is measured. The arm is relaxed with the palm facing the thigh. A measuring tape is placed around the arm, perpendicular to the long axis at the level of the site at with the triceps skinfold is measured. The measurement should not compress the soft tissues and be measured to the nearest 0.1 cm. If the patient is non-ambulatory, the midarm circumference can be measured using either arm while the patient is in the supine position.

Waist Circumference

Waist circumference is predictive of chronic disease (obesity and Type II DM) when the waist measurement is ≥40 inches in men and ≥35 inches in women. Waist circumference should be measured around the person abdomen at the level of the iliac crest.[27-28]

Final Comments Linking Anthropometry to the Next Sections on Diet

Meal rounds can be a continuous quality improvement activity and will allow dietitians to understand more fully the nutrition risk factors in their facility.[29-31]

DIETARY RECOMMENDATIONS

Regular diets should be consistent with the recommendations of the current Dietary Guidelines for Americans (DGA) and the Dietary Reference Intakes, and the recommendations from MyPlate. They address healthy body weight and fitness, following the USDA Food Guide and handling food safely. The textures of regular diets are easily modified for patients needing textural modification and can be converted to low sodium (salt) added diets by omitting salt from the client's tray. House diets contain approximately 2,000 to 2,200 kcals/day. Care must be taken with a regular house diet since it may not meet the needs of all clients; supplemental snacks should be provided for patients with higher energy needs.

The Dietary Guidelines for Americans can be located at the following website: http://www.health.gov/dietaryguidelines/.

The Dietary Reference Intakes can be found at the United States Department of Agriculture's website:https://fnic.nal.usda.gov/.

MyPlate Recommendations can be found at http://www.choosemyplate.gov/.

HOUSE DIETS

REGULAR DIET				
Sample Menu Plan	**Sample Menu**	**Portions**	**Nutrient Content Analysis**	
Breakfast			Energy (kcals)	2154
Whole Grain	Whole Wheat Toast	1 slice	PRO (g [%])	95.72 [17.8]
Whole Grain	Oatmeal	½ cup	CHO (g [%])	309.98 [57.6]
Fruit	Banana	1 med	Total Lipid (g [%])	61.75 [25.8]
Fruit	Orange Juice	½ cup	SFA (g [%])	14.51 [6.1]
Dairy	Fat Free Milk	1 cup	MUFA (g [%])	26.40 [11.0]
Meat	Scrambled Egg Substitute	¼ c raw	PUFA (g [%])	16.25 [6.8]
Oil	Trans-Fat Free Margarine	1 t	Cholesterol (mg)	111
Discretionary Kcals	Jelly	1 T	Fiber (g)	29.6
Beverage	Coffee	As desired[1]	Vitamin A (IU)	30815
			Vitamin E (mg)[2]	7.09
			Vitamin K (mcg)	97.5
Lunch			Vitamin C (mg)	102.5
Whole Grain	Whole Wheat Bun	1 bun	Thiamin (mg)	2.24
Meat	Chicken Breast/canola oil	2 oz/2 t	Riboflavin (mg)	3.00
Vegetable	Lettuce, Shredded	½ cup	Niacin (mg)	27.71
Vegetable	Tomato	2 slices	Pantothenic Acid (mg)	9.56
Other	Yellow mustard	2 t	Vitamin B6 (mg)	2.55
Vegetable	Baked Sweet Potato	½ cup	Folate (mcg)	424
Vegetable	Corn	½ cup	Vitamin B12 (mcg)	6.3
Fruit	Fruit Salad	1 cup	Sodium (mg)	1685
Dairy	Fat Free Milk	1 cup	Potassium (mg)	4821
Oil	Trans-Fat Free Margarine	1 t	Calcium (mg)	1460
Beverage	Iced Tea, Unsweetened	As desired	Iron (mg)	18.29
Dinner			Magnesium (mg)	495
Meat/Oil	Catfish, Baked in canola oil	2½ oz/2 t	Phosphorus (mg)	1820
			Zinc (mg)	11.27
Whole Grain	Brown Rice	½ cup		
Refined Grain	Dinner Roll	1 small		
Vegetable	Black Eyed Peas	½ cup		
Vegetable	Mustard Greens	½ cup		
Fruit	Canned Pineapple	½ cup		
Oil	Trans-Fat Free Margarine	1 t		
Beverage	Iced Tea, Unsweetened	As desired		
Snack				
Grain	Graham Crackers	3		
Fruit	Apple Sauce	½ cup		
Dairy	Fat Free Milk	1 cup		

[1] 1 cup was used in the analysis.
[2] Does not meet the DRI for vitamin E, rotate menus to provide variety in diet or consider supplementation.

HIGH PROTEIN, HIGH ENERGY DIET

INTENDED USE This diet is used when higher intakes of protein and energy are needed. The diet is used to prevent weight loss, tissue wasting, and promote healing. Indications for use include fever, severe burns, excessive weight loss, decubitus ulcers, malnutrition, infection, severe fractures, cancer, and during cancer therapy.

ADEQUACY The high protein, high energy diet meets or exceeds the Dietary Reference Intakes (DRIs) adult males and females. The basic daily food plan for a high protein, high energy diet is not different from a regular house diet. Extra protein can be provided by supplementation or by extra servings of protein rich foods.

RECOMMENDATIONS The high protein, high calorie diet is based on the regular diet with additional servings of high protein, high calorie foods. This diet should provide 100-120 grams of protein, and 3000-4000 kilocalories per day. Three small meals with between-meal feedings provide for better tolerance and acceptance of this diet.

Traditionally, commercial supplements have used to provide additional kilocalories, protein, and other nutrients for elderly in long term facilities[3] and for free-living elderly[4] and they have been shown to be effective in improving nutritional status.[5] However, the elderly may not consume the entire supplement and consumption may interfere with food intake at meals.[3,6-7] Further, study results have been marred by the inconsistent delivery of supplements to all long term residents.[8] Nutrition supplementation with appropriate exercise was also effective in improving the status of the elderly.[9]

Providing an enhanced food program at several meals and increasing the energy density of foods at meals may be satisfactory methods to improve intake in the elderly.[10-11] Increased variety may also increase consumption and improve nutritional status.[12] Further, providing adequate fruit and vegetables also improves the nutritional status of institutionalized elderly.[13] Feeding assistance was also important in improving intake and helping to prevent unintentional weight loss; however, this may be affected by staffing problems.[14-16]

Suggestions for increasing protein and energy intake:

1. Use fortified milk (2 T dry milk powder/cup of fluid milk) for drinking and cooking
2. Use fortified milk to prepare oatmeal, grits, mashed potatoes, puddings, custards, milk shakes, and instant breakfasts
3. Half and half can also be used for cooking or for cereals
4. Snacks should be available so that if the patient is hungry food is available
5. Serve double portions of well-liked foods
6. Add melted margarine or gravy to hot foods
7. Drink fluids away from meals
8. House supplements can be offered; a clear liquid supplement may be better tolerated than a milky one; soups that are supplemental are also available
9. Add corn syrup to fruit ices

10. Add whipped cream to garnish desserts
11. Add cheese to vegetables, grits, and starches
12. Offer higher energy options in every food class--for example, peas in place of string beans, cream soups in place of clear soups
13. Honor food preferences

Although a diet plan with snack foods is presented below, others shown below are available and can be substituted according to the patient's preference and the routine of the nursing and dietary services. Level 1 (least complex)
Milk, whole or 2% are preferred
Ice cream, yogurt, sherbet
Sandwich
Cheese and crackers
Peanut butter and crackers
Pudding, gelatin, custard
100% Fruit Juice

Extra servings of favorite high energy food
 Level 2
House malt, milkshake
Instant breakfast products
Commercial milkshakes

 Level 3
Commercial medical nutritional product

When serving supplements, label each individual supplemental with the individual's complete name, product name, the date, amount, and time of feeding. Cover and chill until served.

Note that this diet exceeds fat and sodium recommendations, and is intended for short term use only.

HIGH PROTEIN HIGH ENERGY DIET

Sample Menu Plan	Sample Menu	Portions	Nutrient Content Analysis	
Breakfast			Energy (kcals)	2863
Whole Grain	Oatmeal	½ c	PRO (g [%])	114.44
Fruit	Banana	1 med	CHO (g [%])	319
Fruit	Apple Juice	½ cup	Total Lipid (g [%])	127.65
Dairy	Whole Milk	1 cup	SFA (g [%])	47.017
Meat	Egg Substitute	¼ cup raw	MUFA (g [%])	48.803
Oil	Trans-Fat Free Margarine	2 t	PUFA (g [%])	28.839
Discretionary Kcals	Jelly	1 T	Cholesterol (mg)	434.00
Beverage	Coffee	1 cup	Fiber (g)	22.9
Mid-Morning Snack			Vitamin A (IU)	30063
Whole Grain	Whole Wheat Toast	1 slice	Vitamin E (mg)	19.28
Fruit	Canned Pineapple	½ cup	Vitamin K (mcg)	175.8
Dairy	Cheese[1]	1 slice	Vitamin C (mg)	120.40
Lunch			Thiamin (mg)	2.02
Whole Grain	Whole Wheat Bun	1 bun	Riboflavin (mg)	3.757
Meat/Oil	Chicken Breast/canola oil	3 oz/ 2 t	Niacin (mg)	29.26
Vegetable	Lettuce, Shredded	½ cup	Pantothenic Acid (mg)	13.693
Vegetable	Tomato	2 slices	Vitamin B6 (mg)	3.106
Other	Mustard	2 t	Folate (mcg)	417.053
Vegetable	Baked Sweet Potato	½ cup	Vitamin B12 (mcg)	7.34
Vegetable	Breen Beans	½ cup	Sodium (mg)	4294
Fruit	Fruit Salad	½ cup	Potassium (mg)	4675
Milk	Whole Milk	1 cup	Calcium (mg)	1954
Oil	Trans-Fat Free Margarine	1T	Iron (mg)	22.28
Beverage	Iced Tea	1 cup	Magnesium (mg)	440
Snack			Phosphorus (mg)	2044
Discretionary Kcals	Fortified Beverage[2]	1 c	Zinc (mg)	17.02
Discretionary Kcals	Graham Crackers	3		
Dinner				
Meat/Oil	Roast Beef/Gravy	2 oz/ 4T		
Refined Grain	Dinner Roll	1 small		
Vegetable	Cream of Potato Soup	1 cup		
Vegetable	Spinach Souffle	½ cup		
Fruit	Mandarin Oranges	½ cupl		
Milk	Whole Milk	1 cup		
Oil	Trans-Fat Free Margarine	2 t		
Beverage	Iced Tea	1 cup		
Snack				
Fruit	Canned Pears	½ c		
Dairy	Custard	½ c		

[1]Cheddar cheese was used in analysis; [2]Ensure was used for analysis; [3]Exceeds fat, SFA, and sodium recommendations and is intended for short term use only.

LIBERALIZED GERIATRIC DIETS

INTENDED USE

Liberalized geriatric diets may be used for healthy or ill older adults in long-term care settings where there is a need for less restrictive dietary modifications for improved intake and meal acceptance. Overly restrictive diets may limit food choices or provide unfamiliar or unpalatable food items for patients with a diminished appetite or taste changes, which may result in inadequate food intake.It is the position of the Academy of Nutrition and Dietetics (AND) that the quality of life and nutritional status of older residents in long-term care facilities may be enhanced by a liberalized diet.[17]

ADEQUACY

Liberalized geriatric diets may meet the Dietary Reference Intakes (DRIs) as established by the Institute of Medicine's Food and Nutrition Board (FNB) for adult males and females. Diets may also exceed the sodium recommendation. Diet modifications are based on the Regular and Modified Consistency Diets listed within this manual. Older individuals may not be able to consume adequate amounts of food and supplementation may be needed.

HOW TO USE THESE DIETS:

1. In a long-term care setting, a liberalized diet allows the older adult to participate in his/her meal decisions and may increase the individual's desire to eat and thereby lessen the risk of malnutrition.

2. To enhance quality of life, individual food habits and food and beverage preferences should be considered in meal planning. Attention to ethnic, cultural, and religious food practices should be honored.

3. If diet modifications are warranted, the least restricted diet is desirable. Stringent diets that limit familiar foods and seasonings may contribute to lower food intake, anxiety, and depression while increasing the risk for weight loss, dehydration, infection, and compromised skin integrity.

4. When planning a nutritionally adequate meal pattern for the older adult, plan three or more meals with a bedtime snack. No more than 14 hours should lapse between the evening meal and the next day's breakfast meal. Bedtime snacks are desirable.

5. The older adult may desire a home-like dining environment. If possible, the individual should eat in a community dining setting rather than in the isolation of a room. This encourages ambulation, increased socialization, and allows for greater assistance and supervision by the attending caregivers. Dining rooms should be pleasant, well lighted, free of offending odors, with avoidable distractions kept to a minimum. Adequate space is to be available allowing the older adult to safely ambulate through the dining area in a wheel chair or walker. Tables that are adjustable to wheel chair height are desired.

19

These amenities may not be possible in acute care facilities.

6. Older adults may experience difficulty in feeding themselves due to a decline in functional ability or dementia. The individual's dining skills may even vary during the day. Although assistance may be needed, every attempt should be made to allow the individual as much independence as possible. Special adaptive feeding utensils and dishware should be considered. An Occupational Therapist is a helpful resource to assess the individual's needs and capabilities. Finger foods may be considered for individuals who can't or won't use eating utensils. Ultimately, however, feeders may be needed to assure maximal intake.

7. Many older adults have difficulty in chewing and swallowing and are at risk of dysphagia. Signs and symptoms of dysphagia include: pocketing of food in the mouth, drooling, wet/gargled voice, coughing or choking on food, and frequent clearing of the throat. Aspiration occurs when foreign material, like liquids and food, enter the lungs via the trachea rather than entering the stomach via the esophagus. Diagnosing dysphagia involves having the individual assessed by a Speech Pathologist. Adjustments in consistency may be recommended after assessment by the Speech Pathologist: chopped, ground and pureed. Modified meat textures should be moist. Liquids also may need consistency change: thickened to the consistency of honey, nectar, or pudding with a special thickening agent. The selected thickening agent should be made with ingredients that allow for maximum release of fluid availability upon digestion (This information can be obtained from the thickener's manufacturer). Correct consistency is critical for the prevention of aspiration and dehydration.

8. With aging, many adults acquire an insensitivity to thirst increasing the individual's risk for dehydration. Fluid needs also increase with fever, nausea, vomiting, diarrhea, and skin wounds. Adequate hydration is critical and involves the caregiver's attention and assistance. Approximately 80% of the available fluids received by an individual in a long-term care setting are received through meals served. Unless the individual is on a physician-ordered fluid restriction, the older adult should have at least 2 beverages (16 oz) served with each meal; water or punch should be available with meals. Between meals, additional fluids should be offered through coffee or punch carts and water pitchers at bedside; thickeners should be used as needed.

9. With aging, sensory loss may occur. Older adults may have lessened abilities to smell and taste foods. Food tastes and appetite may also be affected by medications. Cook foods with more spices and herbs. For many patients, salt added at the table is a possibility and even for patients with salt restrictions, salt at the table may provide less sodium than cooking with salt or using high-sodium processed foods.

10. Constipation may result due to slower digestion with aging, lower fluid intake, and lower intake of fiber. Again, adequate hydration is critical. Unless restricted, include high fiber fruits, vegetables, beans, whole grain cereals and breads, and additional fluids into the meal pattern.

11. If the older individual's meal intake is less than 75%, the caregiver should inquire about the intake and offer an available food item of similar nutritional value as an alternate. Food preferances are also very important. Nutrient-dense supplements (high energy, high protein beverages, puddings, cookies) are also available to use as a meal replacement or between-meal refreshment. The caregiver should monitor the intake of meals and supplements/nourishments to insure that the quantity and volume of these specialized products aren't suppressing meal intake.

FINGER FOOD DIET, REGULAR

INTENDED USE

This diet modification is beneficial to individuals who lack the necessary motor skills to use dining utensils effectively or who, due to memory-related diagnosis, lack the attention or ability to use dining utensils. The diet modification encourages independent dining. Liquids should be served in easy-to-handle mugs or glasses. Older individuals tend to adapt their food to their functional disabilities and it is important to provide a variety of foods.[18] Providing finger foods helps to restore intake and independence in eating and helps maintain weight.[19-20]

ADEQUACY

The regular finger food diet meets the Dietary Reference Intakes (DRIs) as established by the Institute of Medicine's Food and Nutrition Board (FNB) for adult males and females when it is planned following the "Pattern for Daily Food Choices" provided in the Regular Diet section of this manual.

FINGER FOODS	
Breakfast ideas:	***Lunch and Dinner Ideas:***
Cut up fruit slices, *e.g.* orange wedges	Fruit slices drained or piece
Pitted prunes	
Mixed dried fruit	Relish plate-style fresh vegetables: green peppers, sliced
Bacon	tomatoes, cucumbers, carrot sticks, celery sticks, lettuce
Sausage links	pieces, pickles, pitted olives, beets-- can be served with
Hard boiled eggs	dipping sauce
Scrambled egg sandwich	
Other types of breakfast sandwiches	Corn on the cob
Muffins	
Coffee cake	Broccoli, cauliflower and steamed vegetable pieces,
French toast	drained – can be served hot or cold with or without dipping
Graham crackers	sauce
Buttered or dry pancakes	
Buttered or dry waffles	Blenderized soup in a cup
Toast with jelly	
Dry cereal	Sliced dry meats: ham, turkey, beef, cold cuts
Cooked cereal in mug	Pork chops
Biscuits	Chicken pieces: wings, breast, thigh, leg, nuggets—try
Sweet rolls	with dipping sauce
Granola bars	Baked fish, nuggets, or sticks
Pop Tarts	Cheese cubes
	Sauces and gravy in dipping cups
	Hot dog/Hamburger (slice hot dogs length-wise four ways)
	Meat loaf or Salisbury steak
	Sandwiches, wraps, or roll-ups
	Cut up potato pieces, tater tots, French fries, potato chips

	Cornbread, tortillas bread slices, muffins, biscuits, breadsticks, crackers, toast
Beverages Served in mug/glass	*Desserts:* Ice cream bars or Popsicles Smoothies Cake squares, brownies, bar cookies Fruit slices, drained, or pieces Cookies Turnovers Puddings or ice cream served in an ice cream cone

MODIFIED CONSISTENCY DIETS

CLEAR LIQUID DIET

INTENDED USE

The clear liquid diet is intended for short periods of time (not to exceed 3 days) pre-operatively, post-operatively, during acute illnesses, and when it is necessary to minimize the amount of residue in the colon and to maintain hydration in gastrointestinal illness. The clear liquid diet is used to supply fluid, electrolytes, and energy in a form that requires minimal digestion and stimulation of the gastrointestinal tract.

ADEQUACY

This diet is generally inadequate in all essential nutrients and does not meet Dietary Reference Intakes (DRIs) as established by the Institute of Medicine's Food and Nutrition Board (FNB) for adult males and females. This diet exceeds the recommendations for 100% fruit juice. Commercially prepared, low-residue or clear liquid oral supplements can be included, if appropriate for the patient's medical condition. Solid foods, based on appropriate diet prescription, or enteral feeds should be initiated as soon as possible.

RECOMMENDATION Serve 5 or 6 small feedings throughout the day.

CLEAR LIQUID DIET		
Groups	**Foods Allowed**	**Foods to Avoid**
Grains	None	All
Vegetables	None	All
Fruit	Clear juices such as apple, grape, cranberry, or strained juices such as orange juice or grapefruit juice.	All others; any juice with pulp.
Soup	Clear broths, bouillon	All others
Meat, Fish, Poultry, Eggs	None	All
Fats	None	All
Sweets/Desserts	Sugar, honey, syrup, hard sugar candies, plain or flavored gelatin, Popsicles	All others
Beverages	Carbonated/non-carbonated beverages, coffee, tea, fruit-flavored drink mixes made with water	All others
Miscellaneous	Commercial high protein, high energy, clear liquid supplements	All others

CLEAR LIQUID DIET

Sample Plan	Sample Menu	Portion Size	Nutrient Content Without Supplements		Nutrient Content With Supplements	
Breakfast			Energy (kcals)	1201	Energy (kcals)	1951
Fruit	Orange Juice	½ cup	PRO (g [%])	20.9 [7.0]	PRO (g [%])	47.9 [9.8]
Broth/ Bouillon	Strained Beef		CHO (g [%])	272.9 [90.9]	CHO (g [%])	428.9 [87.9]
	Broth	1 cup	Total Lipid (g [%])	2.1 [1.6]	Total Lipid (g [%])	2.1 [1.0]
Other	Strawberry Gelatin	½ cup	SFA (g [%])	0.53 [0.4]	SFA (g [%])	0.53 [0.2]
Beverage	CL Supplement[1]	1 cup	MUFA (g [%])	0.6 [0.5]	MUFA (g [%])	0.6 [0.3]
	Coffee	As desired[2]	PUFA (g [%])	0.56 [0.4]	PUFA (g [%])	0.56 [0.3]
			Cholesterol (mg)	0.0	Cholesterol (mg)	0.0
			Fiber (g)	0.70	Fiber (g)	0.70
Mid-Morning Snack			Vitamin A (IU)	166	Vitamin A (IU)	3916
Fruit	Apple Juice	½ cup	Vitamin E (mg)	1.63	Vitamin E (mg)	28.63
Other	Lime Gelatin	½ cup	Vitamin K (mcg)	7.20	Vitamin K (mcg)	67.20
			Vitamin C (mg)	60.80	Vitamin C (mg)	132.80
Lunch			Thiamin (mg)	0.27	Thiamin (mg)	1.41
Broth/ Bouillon	Chicken Broth	1 cup	Riboflavin (mg)	0.48	Riboflavin (mg)	1.50
Other Fruit	Orange Gelatin	½ cup	Niacin (mg)	1.67	Niacin (mg)	7.67
Beverage	Apple Juice	½ cup	Pantothenic Acid (mg)	1.16	Pantothenic Acid (mg)	3.56
	CL Supplement	1 cup	Vitamin B6 (mg)	0.24	Vitamin B6 (mg)	1.44
	Coffee or Tea	As desired	Folate (mcg)	70	Folate (mcg)	70
			Vitamin B12 (mcg)	0.48	Vitamin B12 (mcg)	4.08
Mid-Afternoon Snack			Sodium (mg)	3434[3]	Sodium (mg)	3569[3]
Fruit	Grape Juice	½ cup	Potassium (mg)	1078	Potassium (mg)	1213
Other	Cherry Gelatin	½ cup	Calcium (mg)	142	Calcium (mg)	292
			Iron (mg)	2.05	Iron (mg)	10.15
Dinner			Magnesium (mg)	99.5	Magnesium (mg)	141.5
Broth/Bouillon	Beef Broth	1 cup	Phosphorus (mg)	398.5	Phosphorus (mg)	1238.5
Other Fruit	Lemon Gelatin	½ cup	Zinc (mg)	0.94	Zinc (mg)	12.34
Beverage	Cranberry Juice	½ cup				
	CL Supplement	1 cup				
	Coffee or Tea	As desired				
Bedtime Snack						
Other	Cherry Popsicle	1 Popsicle				

[1]Abbot Labs clear liquid supplement (Enlive) was used for the nutritional analysis.
[2]1 cup of coffee was used in the analysis.
[3]The sodium content of the diet can be reduced substantially by the use of low sodium chicken and beef broth.

25

FULL LIQUID DIET

INTENDED USE

The Full Liquid Diet is used for a short period post-operatively, during acute illnesses, or when the ability to chew or swallow is severely limited. The diet is limited to foods that are liquid at body temperature. Due to the food restrictions, the diet should not be used for an extended period. Full liquids are considered a transitional diet between clear liquids and solid foods.

ADEQUACY

Because of the elimination of many foods, without supplementation with either commercial supplements or vitamins and minerals, this diet is in certain nutrients required to meet Dietary Reference Intakes (DRIs) as established by the Institute of Medicine's Food and Nutrition Board (FNB) for adult males and females. The nutritional adequacy of the diet can be improved by the addition of high-protein, high energy supplements. The diet is intended for short term use; consider vitamin/mineral supplementation.

RECOMMENDATIONS

1. Between-meal feedings are recommended so that an adequate intake of protein and energy can be obtained.
2. Since milk and dairy products comprise a large portion of this diet, residents who have lactose intolerance may benefit from lactose-reduced or lactose-free products. Those with an allergy to dairy should consume soy formulas or high-protein, high energy supplements as tolerated.

FULL LIQUID DIET			
Groups	**Servings**	**Food Allowed**	**Foods to Avoid**
Grain	5 or more servings	Gruels made from refined cooked cereal.	All others.
Fruits/Vegetables	4 or more servings daily including 1 serving of citrus juice	All strained fruit juice or nectar, vegetable juices, strained or pureed vegetables in soups.	All others.
Dairy	3 cups per day	Milk and milk drinks; lactose-reduced milk products and soy formulas can also be used.	Any containing raw eggs.
Meats	As possible	Pureed meat added to broth or cream soups. Soft cooked or pasteurized egg in eggnogs or custards.	All others. Raw or unpasteurized eggs.
Soups	As desired	Consommés, broths, bouillon, cream soups made from foods allowed.	All others.
Fats	As desired	Butter, margarine, vegetable oils, cream .	All others.
Sweets/Desserts	As desired	Honey, syrups, sugars, custards, gelatins, puddings, ice cream, sherbet (without fruit pulp), fruit ices, Popsicles, yogurt without fruit.	All others.

Beverages	As desired	Coffee, tea, decaffeinated coffee, carbonated, and non-carbonated beverages, fruit-flavored drinks, commercial liquid supplements.	None.
Miscellaneous	As desired	Salt (iodized), flavorings, chocolate, cocoa powder, herbs, spices.	All others.

FULL LIQUID DIET

Sample Menu Plan	Sample Menu	Portion Size	Nutrient Content	
Breakfast			Energy (kcals)	1814
Fruit	Orange Juice	½ cup	PRO (g [%])[2,3]	70.7 [15.6]
Grain	Oatmeal Gruel or Grits	1 cup	CHO (g [%])	288.9 [63.7]
Milk	Choice of Milk	1 cup	Total Lipid (g [%])	44.3 [22.0]
Beverage	Coffee	1 cup	SFA (g [%])	17.8 [8.8]
			MUFA (g [%])	13.1 [6.5]
Mid-Morning Snack			PUFA (g [%])	9.5 [4.7]
Fruit	Grape Juice	½ cup	Cholesterol (mg)	272
Desserts	Fortified Pudding	½ cup	Fiber (g)	10.1
			Vitamin A (IU)	9837
Lunch			Vitamin E (mg)	10.32
Vegetable/Soup	Cream of Potato Soup with Pureed Potatoes	1 cup	Vitamin K (mcg)	52.6
			Vitamin C (mg)	101.5
Juice	Apple Juice	½ cup	Thiamin (mg)	1.575
Dessert	Strawberry Gelatin	½ cup	Riboflavin (mg)	3.091
Beverage	Eggnog	½ cup	Niacin (mg)	14.49
	Coffee/Tea	1 cup	Pantothenic Acid (mg)	11.62
			Vitamin B6 (mg)	1.588
Mid-Afternoon Snack			Folate (mcg)	331.5
Sweets/Desserts	Fortified Beverage (Commercial Supplement)	1 cup	Vitamin B12 (mcg)	6.42
			Sodium (mg)	2529
			Potassium (mg)	3580
Dinner			Calcium (mg)	1566
Fruit	Pineapple Juice	½ cup	Iron (mg)	12.97
	Vegetable Soup with	1 cup	Magnesium (mg)	390
Vegetable/ Soup	Pureed Vegetables		Phosphorus (mg)	1686
Dairy	Baked Custard	½ cup	Zinc (mg)	15.4
	Choice of Milk	1 cup		
	Coffee/Tea	1 cup		
Bedtime Snack				
Dairy	Vanilla Ice Cream	½ cup		

MECHANICALLY ALTERED DIETS

INTENDED USE

The Mechanically Altered Diets are used when an individual has difficulty chewing or experiences dysphagia. Foods should be mechanically altered by chopping, grinding, or pureeing foods with a food processor so they are easier and safer to swallow. An evaluation team consisting of the physician, licensed dietitian/nutritionist, speech pathologist, or occupational therapist, and nurse can determine the consistency of food that is appropriate.

One of the following modified diets should be ordered after the evaluation:

Chewing Problems: Pureed or Chopped (Mechanical/Dental Soft). This can be a regular diet or any type of therapeutic diet.

Swallowing Problems:

National Dysphagia Diet I (NDD): Dysphagia-Pureed (homogenous, very cohesive, pudding-like, requiring very little chewing ability).

National Dysphagia Diet II: Dysphagia-Mechanical Altered (cohesive, moist, semisolid foods, requiring some chewing).

National Dysphagia Diet III: Dysphagia-Advanced (soft foods that require more chewing ability).

Level	Foods Allowed	Foods Not Allowed
Level I	Pudding-like foods with a smooth consistency with no lumps.	Fruited yogurt, gelatin, peanut butter, scrambled, fried, or hard-boiled eggs, unblenderized cottage cheese
Level II	Moist and soft-textured foods including tender ground and finely diced meat, soft cooked vegetables, soft fruit (including canned) and some cereals that have been moistened.	Corn, peas, cubed cheese, rice, bread, and cake.
Level III	Most regular foods except those items which are overly hard, crunchy, or sticky.	Hard foods like hard raw vegetables and fruits, corn skins, nuts, and seeds.

ADEQUACY

These diets may meet the Dietary Reference Intakes (DRIs) as established by the Institute of Medicine's Food and Nutrition Board (FNB) for adult males and females if a wide variety of foods are selected and adequate quantities are consumed; however, studies have shown that pureed diets may be low in protein.[21] The menus may not meet the MyPlate recommendations for whole grains or the DRI for fiber, since chewing whole grain foods may be difficult. Oral supplements may be used to meet nutritional needs. Alternately, pureed foods may be supplemented with vitamins and minerals.[22] In addition, since any therapeutic diet can be converted to a mechanical soft diet, there is the possibly that the initial diet, for example a renal diet may not meet the DRIs.

RECOMMENDATIONS

1. Plan menus that have eye and flavor appeal.
2. Pureed foods should be served separately so that each food will retain its distinct flavor and taste. Do not combine meat, vegetable, and starch in one dish.
3. Commercial stabilizers can be used to make foods easier for people with dysphagia to swallow. Foods that are too thin and thin liquids are difficult to swallow.
4. Soft foods with high acceptability for individuals with chewing problems include: soft breads, finely ground or chopped meats served with broth or gravy, cooked vegetables, and fruits that are tender and do not have tough skins.
5. Some combinations of foods that are well accepted include:
   a. Pureed egg or soft cooked egg with cooked cereal.
   b. Pureed meats stabilized with instant mashed potatoes, cooked oatmeal, or commercial stabilizers.
   c. Non-fat dry milk added to cooked products such as potatoes, gravies, soups, sauces, and puddings to increase protein.
   d. Bran cereal added to cooked cereals.
   e. Liquid oil or margarine added to foods to increase kilocalories.
6. For dysphagia diets, avoid foods that crumble and fall apart easily, such as dry crumbly breads, crackers, plain rice, and plain ground meats.

> **Any type of diet can be converted to a dental soft diet or to a mechanically altered diet. Dysphagia diets may need to be modified with specific foods for specific textures.**

PUREED DIET

PURPOSE
The pureed diet is designed for alert individuals who have difficulty chewing/swallowing and do not tolerate a chopped (mechanical/dental soft) diet such as in cases of stroke, poor detention, oral surgery, oral or esophageal cancer, or esophageal stricture.

DESCRIPTION
The diet consists of regular foods that are blenderized or strained and liquids (pureed, homogenous, and cohesive). It may be modified for other therapeutic regimens, *e.g.* fat, protein, or carbohydrate controlled, as appropriate. Foods should have a smooth pudding-like consistency.

ADEQUACY
These diets may meet the Dietary Reference Intakes (DRIs) as established by the Institute of Medicine's Food and Nutrition Board (FNB) for adult males and females if a wide variety of foods are selected and adequate quantitied are consumed; however, studies have shown that pureed diets may be low in protein.[21] In addition, it may be difficult to meet the recommendations for fiber, folate, and other nutrients associated with grains.

Food Group	Foods Allowed	Foods Not Allowed
Grains	Cooked cereal without fruit or nuts; mashed or creamed potatoes; pureed rice or noodles thinned with a sauce	Dry cereal, cooked cereal with fruit and nuts; all breads; sweet potatoes
Fruit	Fruit juices and nectars, fruit drinks, pureed fruits without seeds or large chunks	All others
Vegetables	Vegetable juices, pureed cooked vegetables without seeds	All others
Dairy	Milk, plain yogurt, milkshakes, malts	None
Meat and Meat Alternates	Strained or pureed meat, fish and poultry; pureed cottage cheese, cheese sauce; soft poached, scrambled or boiled eggs; egg substitutes	Whole meats, fish or poultry; hard cooked or fried eggs
Soups	Broth, bouillon, consommé, soups with pureed vegetables, strained cream soups	All others
Fats and Oils	Margarine, oil, cream, cream substitutes, gravies, cream sauces, whipped topping	All others

Desserts	Gelatin, plain custard or pudding, ice cream, ice milk, sherbet, flavored fruit ices, Popsicles, fruit whips, plain Bavarian creams	Any made with coconut, nuts, or whole fruit
Beverages	Coffee, decaffeinated coffee, tea, and carbonated beverages	Any not tolerated; alcohol
Miscellaneous Condiments	Catsup, mustard, vinegar	Horseradish, chili sauce, olives, pickles, seeds
Seasonings	Salt, pepper, powdered herbs and spices	All others
Sweets	Sugar, syrup, honey, jelly, chocolate syrup	Jams, preserves, candy

PUREED DIET

Sample Menu Plan	Sample Menu	Portion Size	Nutrient Content	
Breakfast			Energy (kcals)	2336[2]
Grain	Cream of Wheat	½ cup	PRO (g [%])	110.4 [19]
Grain	Pureed Bread	1slice	CHO (g [%])	246.98 [43]
Fruit	Orange Juice	½ cup	Total Lipid (g [%])	102.39 [39][3]
Meat/ Meat Alternate	Pureed or very soft cooked or poached egg	1	SFA (g [%])	32.74 [12]
			MUFA (g [%])	39.79 [15]
Fat	Margarine	2 t	PUFA (g [%])	20.532 [8]
Milk	Choice of Milk[1]	1 cup	Cholesterol (mg)	489.00[4]
Beverage	Coffee	1 cup	Fiber (g)	23.1
Lunch			Vitamin A (IU)	40125
			Vitamin E (mg)	14.54
Meat or Meat	Pureed Baked Chicken in	2oz	Vitamin K (mcg)	530.5
Alternate	Natural Gravy	¼ cup	Vitamin C (mg)	93.40
Grain	Steamed Rice, Pureed	½ cup	Thiamin (mg)	1.50
Grain	Pureed Bread	1 slice	Riboflavin (mg)	2.92
Vegetable	Pureed Sweet Potatoes	½ cup	Niacin (mg)	27.90
Vegetable	Pureed String Beans	½ cup	Pantothenic Acid (mg)	7.99
Fat	Margarine	2 t	Vitamin B6 (mg)	2.46
Beverage	Choice of Milk	1 cup	Folate (mcg)	365.34
	Iced Tea	1 cup	Vitamin B12 (mcg)	10.57
Afternoon Snack			Sodium (mg)	2681[5]
			Potassium (mg)	3347
Fruit	Pureed Bananas	1 medium	Calcium (mg)	1107.9
Dinner			Iron (mg)	79.44
			Magnesium (mg)	850
Meat/Beans	Pureed Ground Beef in	3 oz	Phosphorus (mg)	1189.79
	Natural Gravy	¼ cup	Zinc (mg)	6.85
Grain	Pureed Bread	1 slice		
Vegetable	Vegetable Soup with Pureed	½ cup		
Vegetable	Vegetables	1 cup		
Fruit	Pureed Canned Pears	½ cup		
Fat	Margarine	2 t		
Beverage	Iced Tea	1 cup		
Bedtime Snack				
Fruit	Apple Juice	½ cup		
Dessert/Milk	Custard	½ cup		

[1]Milk choice depends on the patient's need for energy and the presence of any concomitant disease such as heart disease. For the nutrient analysis, fat-free milk was used; if additional energy is needed, whole milk can be used.
[2]If energy exceeds estimated needs, reduce the serving size of foods, or substitute a pureed vegetable for the soup at dinner.
[3]This exceeds the recommendations for fat; for the analysis, 80/20 ground meat was used; a leaner version can be used and the amount of margarine can be reduced. Custard could also be prepared with fat-free milk.
[4]The egg, custard, and ground beef contribute to the cholesterol level of this menu; egg substitute can be used at breakfast and in the custard to lower the cholesterol level of the menu.
[5]The sodium content can be reduced by using home-prepared gravies rather than commercial ones.

CHOPPED DIET (MECHANICAL SOFT)

PURPOSE
The chopped diet is designed for alert individuals who have chewing difficulties requiring modification in texture to minimize the amount of chewing necessary for ingestion of food.

DESCRIPTION
The diet contains all foods from the regular diet as well as chopped or ground foods. Patients may tolerate ground turkey better than ground beef. Soft well cooked vegetables with less than ½ inch pieces are allowed except for corn, peas, and other specific fibrous varieties.The diet must be individualized according to tolerance and acceptance. If the original menu meets the dietary recommendations, the mechanical soft version will meet the requirements.

ADEQUACY
Any regular or therapeutic diet can be converted to a mechanical soft (dental soft) diet; thus the nutrition adequacy of the diet depends on the nutritional adequacy of the original diet. Although many of the diets in this manual meet the DRIs set by the IOM FNB, not all can. It patients have trouble chewing whole grains, they may not be able to meet the MyPlate recommendations for grains. Softer whole grains, such as oatmeal can be included in the diet, but coarser products like some breaks may not be suitable.

MECHANICAL SOFT DIET

Sample Menu Plan	Sample Menu	Portion Size	Nutrient Analysis	
Breakfast			Energy (kcals)	2305
Grain	White Bread	1slice	PRO (g [%])	96.78 [17]
Grain	Oatmeal	½ cup	CHO (g [%])	271.85 [47]
Fruit	Orange Juice	½ cup	Total Lipid (g [%])	93.72 [36]
Fruit	Banana	1medium	SFA (g [%])	29.769 [11]
Milk	Fat-free Milk	1cup	MUFA (g [%])	35.906 [14]
Meat	Scrambled Egg Substitute	¼ cup raw	PUFA (g [%])	19.561 [8]
Fat	Margarine	2t	Cholesterol (mg)	258
Beverage	Coffee	As desired[1]	Fiber (g)	18.9
Lunch			Vitamin A (IU)	26956
Meat & Beans	Chopped Stewed Chicken	2 oz	Vitamin E (mg)	12.07
Grain	Soft Dinner Roll	1 roll	Vitamin K (mcg)	147.3
Grain	Steamed Rice	½ cup	Vitamin C (mg)	134
Vegetables	Swett Potatoes	½ cup	Thiamin (mg)	1.777
Vegetables	Chopped Steamed Cabbage	½ cup	Riboflavin (mg)	2.866
Fruit	Canned Fruit Salad	½ cup	Niacin (mg)	26.684
Fat	Gravy	2 oz	Pantothenic Acid (mg)	9.138
Fat	Margarine	2 t	Vitamin B6 (mg)	2.523
Milk	Fat-free Milk	1 cup	Folate (mcg)	272.053
Beverage	Iced Tea	As desired	Vitamin B12 (mcg)	6.1
Dinner			Sodium (mg)	2211
Meat/ Beans	Ground beef[2]	3 oz	Potassium (mg)	3899
Grain	White bread	1 slice	Calcium (mg)	1182
Vegetables	String beans	½ cup	Iron (mg)	19.68
Fruit	Canned Mandarin Oranges	½ cup	Magnesium (mg)	310
Fat	Margarine	2 t	Phosphorus (mg)	1494
Fat	Gravy	2 oz	Zinc (mg)	13.98
Beverage	Iced Tea	As desired		
Dessert	Cherry Gelatin	½ cup		
Bedtime Snack				
Milk	Custard	½ cup		
Fruit	Canned Pears	½ cup		

[1]One cup was used in the analysis.
[2] Some individuals find ground turkey softer to chew than ground beef.

DYSPHAGIA DIETS[23]

PURPOSE
Dysphagia diets are designed to provide foods which are safe and easy to swallow. Dysphagia connotes a disturbance in the normal transfer of food from the oral cavity to the stomach and refers to the difficulty in swallowing liquids, solids, or both. This swallowing disability may be the result of such conditions as stroke, head injury, cerebral palsy, Parkinson's disease, other neuromuscular diseases, and head or neck cancer. Dysphagia Diets are designed to: 1) reduce the risks associated with choking and gagging; 2) reduce the risk of aspiration; and 3) stimulate re-establishment of the swallow reflex.

Warning Signs of Swallowing Problems

- Coughing while eating or drinking or very soon after eating or drinking.
- "Wet" or "gurgly" voice, especially after eating.
- Holding or pocketing food in mouth.
- Drooling or losing food at corner of mouth.
- Spitting food out of mouth/tongue thrusting.
- Slow eating.
- Not eating.
- Multiple swallows on a single mouthful of food.
- Obvious extra effort or difficulty while chewing or swallowing.
- Inadequate intake of food or fluid.
- Unexplained weight loss.
- Repetitive pneumonia
- Facial Weakness
- Slurred Speech
- Frequent throat clearing

NOTES: Some persons with dysphagia can aspirate silently without showing any of the above signs. In acute care facilities, the number of patients with dysphagia has increased since 2000 and is age dependent; thus, it is important to also assess patients in long-term care facilities for dysphagia.[22]

Dysphagia I Diet

Rationale: This diet is designed for patients who need axmimum restriction due to dysphagia and inability to swallow chewable foods. Foods that are sticky or require bolus formation or controlled manipulation in the mouth (*i.e.,* melted cheese, peanut butter) are omitted.

Description: Thick pureed foods with smooth textures are used. Liquids are thickened to desired consistency, as needed, with a commercial thickening agent.

Foods Allowed and not Allowed on Dysphagia Diets		
Group	**Foods Allowed**	**Foods Not Allowed**
Grains	Plain cooked cereal; mashed potatoes; pureed rice or pasta; pureed cream corn	Hard breads; French toast; potato peel; whole kernel corn; bread; crackers; pancakes; cold cereal, unless softened with commercial thickening agent or gelatin
Fruit	Pureed fruits without seeds or large chunks; applesauce or pureed pineapple with thickener; thickened fruit juices and nectars	Fruits with seeds or fruits- whole or pieces; citrus fruits
Vegetables	Pureed cooked vegetables; tossed salad pureed and thickened; thickened vegetable juices	All other raw vegetables; cooked vegetables- whole or pieces
Dairy	Smooth yogurt (*e.g.* no fruit pieces, nuts), thickened milk, milk shakes, thickened liquid supplements	Other milk products
Meat and Meat Alternates	Pureed meat, fish, or poultry; pureed cottage cheese; cheese sauce; pureed cooked eggs or egg substitute	Whole meats, fish, or poultry, hard cooked or fried eggs; peanut butter
Soups	Smooth cream soups; thickened broth; pureed and thickened soups	All others
Fats and Oils	Margarine, oil, gravies, cream, cream substitutes, cream sauces, whipped topping, mayonnaise	All others
Desserts	Plain custard or pudding; smooth pie filling	Any dessert with coconut, nuts, raisins, or whole fruit; plain cakes and cookies, unless softened with commercial thickening agent or gelatin; ice cream, sherbet or gelatin, unless thin liquids are allowed.
Beverages	Thickened; fruit drinks, coffee, tea, water, carbonated beverages	All thin liquids
Condiments	Ketchup, mustard	Any containing seeds, nuts, or relish
Seasoning	Salt, pepper, powdered herbs and spices	Herbs and spices with seeds
Sweets	Sugar, syrup, honey, jelly	Jams, preserves, candy

DYSPHAGIA I DIET

Sample Plan	Sample Menu	Portion Size	Nutrient Content	
Breakfast			Energy (kcals)	2454
Fruit	Orange Juice, thickened	½ cup	PRO (g [%])	109.33
Grain	Oatmeal	½ cup	CHO (g [%])	273.92
Grain	Softened Bread	1 slice	Total Lipid (g [%])	104.52
Meat	Pureed egg substitute	¼ cup raw	SFA (g [%])	30.695
Fat	Margarine	1 t	MUFA (g [%])	40.478
Milk	Skim Milk, thickened	1 cup	PUFA (g [%])	24.193
Beverage	Coffee, thickened	1 cup	Cholesterol (mg)	268.00
Mid-Morning Snack			Fiber (g)	23.9
			Vitamin A (IU)	38606
Fruit	Banana, pureed	1 med	Vitamin E (mg)	24.24
Lunch			Vitamin K (mcg)	680.2
Meat or Beans	Pureed Baked Chicken in Broth	2 oz.	Vitamin C (mg)	147.20
Grain	Pureed Steamed Rice	⅓ cup	Thiamin (mg)	2.711
Grain	Softened Dinner Roll	1 roll	Riboflavin (mg)	3.281
Vegetable	Pureed Green Beans	½ cup	Niacin (mg)	30.546
Vegetable	Pureed Sweet Potatoes	½ cup	Pantothenic Acid (mg)	11.424
Fruit	Canned Fruit Salad	½ cup	Vitamin B6 (mg)	2.978
Fat	Margarine	2 t	Folate (mcg)	468
Fat	Natural Gravy, thickened	4 T	Vitamin B12 (mcg)	7.59
Dairy	Skim Milk, thickened	1 cup	Sodium (mg)	2403
Mid-Afternoon Snack			Potassium (mg)	4389
Discretionary Kcals	Fortified Beverage[2]	1 cup	Calcium (mg)	1590
			Iron (mg)	24.73
Dinner			Magnesium (mg)	465
Meat or Beans	Ground Beef, pureed	3 oz.	Phosphorus (mg)	1773
Grain	Softened Bread	1 slice	Zinc (mg)	17.75
Vegetable	Pureed Spinach	½ cup		
Vegetable	Pureed Steamed Cabbage	½ cup		
Milk	Fat-Free Milk, thickened	1 cup		
Fat	Margarine	2t		
Bedtime Snack				
Fruit	Canned Pears, pured	½ cup		
Milk	Custard	½ cup		

[1]Nutrient analysis was performed without the energy/carbohydrate content of the thickening agent. When thickened to a spoon-thick consistency, dysphagia diets have been shown to reduce the risk of aspiration in stroke patients (44). Whole milk or starchy vegetables can be used to increase energy intake if needed.
[2]Ensure was used in the nutrient analysis—thicken as needed.

DYSPHAGIA II DIET

RATIONALE

This diet is designed for individuals who may have difficulty chewing, manipulating, and swallowing certain foods. It consists of soft food items prepared with a minimum of pureeing. It may be appropriate for persons beginning to chew or with mild oral preparatory stage deficits.

DESCRIPTION

Textures are soft with no tough skins, nuts or dry, chewy, crispy, raw, or stringy foods are allowed. Meats should be ground with gravy. Liquids may be thickened as needed.

Food Group	Foods Allowed	Foods Not Allowed
Grain	Plain cooked cereal; mashed potatoes; pureed rice bit sized noodles or pasta with sauce or gravy.	Hard breads; potato peel; whole kernel corn; bread; crackers; pancakes; cold cereal, unless softened with commercial thickening agent or gelatin
Fruit	Chopped soft fresh fruit and canned fruit without seeds, seeds or tough fibers; applesauce or pureed pineapple with thickener; pureed honeydew or cantaloupe; and fruit juices and nectars*	Whole fruits; hard fresh fruits (apple, honeydew, cantaloupe); citrus fruits
Vegetables	Bite-sized cooked vegetables; tossed salad pureed and thickened, vegetable juices.*	All other raw vegetables; whole cooked vegetables; broccoli stems; molded vegetable salads
Dairy	Milk.* Yogurt milk shakes, liquid supplements.*	Other milk products
Meat and Meat Alternates	Meat ground with a medium to thick gravy that holds together; cottage cheese; meat salads with minced ingredients; bite size casseroles; scrambled, fried or poached egg or egg substitute	Whole meats, fish, or poultry, hard cooked or fried eggs; peanut butter
Soups	Cream soups; broth.* Bite-sized vegetables and noodle soups	Soups with chunks of meat or vegetables
Fats and Oils	Margarine, oil, gravies, cream, cream substitutes, cream sauces, whipped topping, mayonnaise	All others
Desserts	Plain custard or pudding; smooth pie filling; bread pudding without raisins; gelatin;* ice cream;* sherbet;* fruit ices*	Any dessert with coconut, nuts, raisins, or whole fruit; plain cakes and cookies, unless softened with commercial thickening agent or gelatin
Beverages	Fruit drinks, coffee, tea, water, carbonated beverages	Refer to list of dysphagia thin/thick liquids. Serve according to individual needs
Condiments	Ketchup, mustard	Any containing seeds, nuts, or relish
Seasoning	Salt, pepper, powdered herbs and spices	Herbs and spices with seeds
Sweets	Sugar, syrup, honey, jelly	Jams, preserves, candy
*If thickened liquids are needed, refer to list of dysphagia thin/thick liquids.		

DYSPHAGIA II DIET				
Sample Menu Plan	Sample Menu	Portion Size	Nutrient Content[1]	
Breakfast			Energy (kcals)	1976
Grain	Oatmeal	½ cup	PRO (g [%])	91.79 [19]
Grain	Plain Bread, softened	1 slice	CHO (g [%])	235.07 [48]
Fruit	Apple Juice*	½ cup	Total Lipid (g [%])	74.23 [34]
Meat and Beans	Egg Substitute	¼ cup raw	SFA (g [%])	24.485 [11][2]
			MUFA (g [%])	30.933 [14]
Milk	Fat-Free Milk*	1 cup	PUFA (g [%])	19.735 [9]
Fat	Margarine	2 t	Cholesterol (mg)	321.00
Beverage	Coffee*	1 cup	Fiber (g)	17.7
Lunch			Vitamin A (IU)	36531
Meat and Beans/Fat	Ground Roast Beef in Gravy	2 oz./ 4T	Vitamin E (mg)	12.16
			Vitamin K (mcg)	564.8
Vegetable	Steamed Cabbage, chopped	½ cup	Vitamin C (mg)	41.30
Vegetable	Sweet Potatoes, chopped	½ cup	Thiamin (mg)	2.349
Grain	Pureed Rice	½ cup	Riboflavin (mg)	2.976
Grain	Softened Bread	1 slice	Niacin (mg)	24.922
Fat	Margarine	2 t	Pantothenic Acid (mg)	8.948
Dessert	Custard	½ cup	Vitamin B6 (mg)	2.166
Beverage	Iced Tea	1 cup	Folate (mcg)	298
Dinner			Vitamin B12 (mcg)	5.21
Meat or Meat Alternate	Ground Baked Chicken in Gravy	2 oz./4 T	Sodium (mg)	2136
Grain	Softened Bread	1 slice	Potassium (mg)	3599
Vegetable	Mashed Potatoes	½ cup	Calcium (mg)	1421
Vegetable	Green Beans, chopped	½ cup	Iron (mg)	18.63
Vegetable	Spinach, chopped	½ cup	Magnesium (mg)	349
Fruit	Fruit Cocktail, chopped	½ cup	Phosphorus (mg)	1508
Fat	Margarine	2t	Zinc (mg)	9.97
Milk	Fat-Free Milk*	1 cup		
Bedtime Snack				
Fruit	Canned Pears, chopped	½ cup		
Milk	Eggnog	½ cup		

[1]Nutrient analysis was performed without the energy/carbohydrate content of the thickening agent.
[2] This menu exceeds the saturdated fatty acid recommendations; if the patient has risk factors for cardiovascular disease, the eggnog can be replaced by fat-free milk.
*If thickened liquids are needed, refer to list of dysphagia thin/thick liquids.

DYSPHAGIA III DIET

RATIONALE
This diet is designed for individuals who chew soft textures. The diet is based on a mechanical soft (chopped) diet and may be appropriate for persons with mild oral preparatory stage deficits.

DESCRIPTION
Foods are soft and in bite-size pieces. Meats are minced unless otherwise specified. No nuts are allowed.

Group	Foods Allowed	Foods Not Allowed
Grain	Cooked cereal; dry cereal,* mashed potatoes; rice with gravy,* noodles, or pasta; soft bread; pancakes; French toast	Hard breads such as bagel, cereal with nuts
Fruit	Chopped soft fresh fruits and canned fruits; 100% fruit juices and nectars*	Hard fresh fruits
Vegetables	All cooked vegetables soft and bite sized; chopped salads and raw vegetables, vegetable juices*	Whole, raw, or cooked vegetables (al dente)
Dairy	All milk products.*	Yogurt with nuts or coconut
Meat and Meat Alternates	Minced meats; chopped fish; bite-sized meat casseroles; cottage cheese; egg or egg substitute; creamy peanut butter	Whole meats, fish, or poultry, hard cooked or fried eggs; chunky peanut butter
Soups	Any, except those under not allowed	Any nuts
Fats and Oils	Margarine, oil, gravies, cream, cream substitutes, cream sauces, whipped topping, mayonnaise	All others
Desserts	Any except those under not allowed	Any dessert with nuts
Beverages	Fruit drinks,* coffee,* tea,* water,* carbonated beverages*	Refer to list of dysphagia thin/thick liquids. Serve according to individual needs
Condiments	As allowed	None
Seasoning	As allowed	None
Sweets	As allowed	None
*If thickened liquids are needed, refer to list of dysphagia thin/thick liquids.		

DYSPHAGIA III DIET				
Sample Menu Plan	**Sample Menu**	**Portion Size**	**Nutrient Content**[1]	
Breakfast			Energy (kcals)	1976
Grain	Oatmeal	½ cup	PRO (g [%])	91.79 [19]
Grain	Plain Bread	1 slice	CHO (g [%])	235.07 [48]
Fruit	Apple Juice*	½ cup	Total Lipid (g [%])	74.23 [34]
Meat and Beans	Egg Substitute	¼ cup raw	SFA (g [%])	24.485 [11][2]
Milk	Fat-Free Milk*	1 cup	MUFA (g [%])	30.933 [14]
Fat	Margarine	2 t	PUFA (g [%])	19.735 [9]
Beverage	Coffee*	1 cup	Cholesterol (mg)	321.00
Lunch			Fiber (g)	17.7
Meat and Beans/Fat	Ground Roast Beef in Gravy	2 oz/4T	Vitamin A (IU)	36531
Grain	Rice	½ cup	Vitamin E (mg)	12.16
Grain	Bread	1 slice	Vitamin K (mcg)	564.8
Vegetable	Steamed Cabbage, chopped	½ cup	Vitamin C (mg)	41.30
Vegetable	Sweet Potatoes, chopped	½ cup	Thiamin (mg)	2.349
Fat	Margarine	2 t	Riboflavin (mg)	2.976
Dessert	Custard	½ cup	Niacin (mg)	24.922
Beverage	Iced Tea*	1 cup	Pantothenic Acid (mg)	8.948
Supper			Vitamin B6 (mg)	2.166
Meat or Meat Alternate	Ground Baked Chicken in Gravy	2 oz./4T	Folate (mcg)	298
			Vitamin B12 (mcg)	5.21
Grain	Mashed Potatoes	1 slice	Sodium (mg)	2136
Vegetable	Green Beans, chopped	½ cup	Potassium (mg)	3599
Vegetable	Spinach, chopped	½ cup	Calcium (mg)	1421
Fruist	Fruit Cocktail	½ cup	Iron (mg)	18.63
Fat	Margarine	2 t	Magnesium (mg)	349
Milk	Fat-Free Milk*	1 cup	Phosphorus (mg)	1508
Bedtime Snack			Zinc (mg)	9.97
Fruit	Canned Pears	½ cup		
Milk	Eggnog	½ cup		

[1]Nutrient analysis was performed without the energy/carbohydrate content of the thickening agent.

[2]This menu exceeds the saturated fatty acid recommendations; if the patient has risk factors for cardiovascular disease, the eggnog can be replaced by fat-free milk.

*If thickened liquids are needed, refer to list of dysphagia thin/thick liquids.

DYSPHAGIA DIET LIQUID CONSISTENCIES

Liquids may pose a particular problem for patients with dysphagia, so it is very important to determine the type of liquid that is safe for each individual to swallow. Thin liquids are usually the most difficult to swallow. Thickening liquids slows the time it takes for fluid to move through the mouth and esophagus, allows better control of the swallow, and decreases risk of aspiration pneumonia. Liquids can be thickened by commercial starch or gum based products like Thicken Up, Thick & Easy, Thik & Clear, and Simply Thick.

General Guidelines for Restriction of Thin Liquids:

1. No iced beverages.
2. Avoid soup unless pureed and thickened.
3. No cold cereal, unless softened with thickened liquid.
4. Foods that are liquid at room temperature should be avoided, such as ice cream, sherbet, gelatins.
5. Do not serve fruits and vegetables with high liquid content, such as tomatoes, citrus sections, pineapple, or watermelon.
6. All fruits and vegetables should be drained to remove excess liquid.
7. If no specific level of liquid consistency is ordered, use "honey consistency."
8. When thickening liquids, follow instructions provided by commercial thickening products for proportions of thickener and liquids to achieve desired liquid consistency.

EXAMPLES OF LIQUID CONSISTENCIES

THIN LIQUIDS (Most Difficult to Swallow)- regular liquids, no adjustments

Water	Ices
Tea	Plain gelatin
Coffee	Commercial Supplements
Broth	Ice Cream
Fruit Juices	Frozen Yogurt
Soft Drinks	Thin Vegetable Juices
Milk	

NECTAR OR SYRUP CONSISTENCY LIQUIDS – falls slowly from a spoon and can be sipped through a straw or from a cup

Vegetable Juice
Fruit Nectars
Cream Soups
Buttermilk
Milk Shakes (without thickeners)
Liquids thickened with Commercial Products
Thickened Commercial Supplements

HONEY CONSISTENCY – drops from a spoon, but too thick to sipped through a straw
Honey Like liquids are thickened to honey consistency by using commercial thickeners.
Thick Cream Soups
Thick Milk Shakes
Thick Eggnog_
Tomato sauce

SPOON-THICK LIQUIDS OR PUDDING CONSISTENCY – maintains shape, needs to be eaten with a spoon, too thick to drink
Commercial thickening agents are needed to thicken liquids to a pudding consistency

It is difficult to achieve hydration at this level of thickness because the flavor and mouth-feel of the original liquid may be greatly diminished, making it less attractive to the patient.

Dysphagia-Diet.com also provides resources for dietitians.[23]

REDUCED SODIUM DIET

INTENDED USE
This diet is used in the treatment of congestive heart failure,[1-7] some kidney diseases,[8-13] and ascites from cirrhosis of the liver or other dieases.[14-19] Patients and their families should be instructed on label reading, not using salt at the table, and cooking techniques to provide tasty food without salt. Patients who traditionally followed a basic reduced sodium diet to treat hypertension should be counseled to follow the DASH diet (Dietary Approaches to Stop Hypertension). [20]

ADEQUACY
These diets are adequate and meet the Dietary Reference Intakes (DRIs) as established by the Institute of Medicine's Food and Nutrition Board (FNB) for adult males and females. The sample menu here also provides ~ 2000 kcals per day and meets MyPlate recommendations for food groups.

GENERAL DESCRIPTION The 2 gm sodium diet restricts the use of foods prepared with salt or served with salt. All foods with high sodium contents are omitted.

General Guidelines:

1. Do not use salt in food preparation or at the table.
2. Avoid all cured, canned, or smoked meats.
3. Avoid instant or quick-cook products.
4. Avoid canned and instant soups, stews, chili, and bouillon cubes, unless products are low sodium.
5. Consult a physician if the patient wishes to use salt substitutes.

Shopping and cooking tips:

- Salt is often added to foods during processing.
- Some sodium containing ingredients include:
  - Salt (NaCl)
  - Sodium Saccharin
  - Sodium (Na)
  - Sodium nitrate
  - Brine (salt and water)
  - Sodium proprionate
  - Monosodium glutamate (MSG)
  - Any ingredient with sodium in its name
  - Sodium Bicarbonate (baking soda)

SODIUM CLAIMS ON FOOD LABELS:

- Sodium Free
  - Less than 5 mg sodium per serving
- Salt free
  - Meets requirements for sodium free
- Low sodium
  - 140 mg sodium or less per serving
- Very low sodium
  - 35 mg or less sodium per serving
- Reduced Sodium
  - At least 25% less sodium when compared with the regular version of that product.
- Light in sodium
  - 50% less sodium per serving, restricted to foods with more than 40 calories per serving or more than 3 g of fat per serving (if pertaining to sodium content)
- Unsalted, without added salt, No salt added
  - No salt is added during processing
  - Salt substitutes

Food Group	Choose More Often	Avoid
Grains	Whole grain products, *e.g.* bulgur wheat, unsalted popcorn, whole grain breads, rolls; pasta; enriched grain products; muffins, cornbread, and waffles; most dry cereals, cooked cereal without added salt; unsalted crackers and breadsticks.	Breads, rolls, and crackers with salted tops; quick breads; instant hot cereals; pancakes; commercial bread stuffing and pasta mixes; self-rising flour and biscuit mixes.
Vegetables	Fresh, frozen, or low sodium canned vegetables or vegetable juices; low sodium tomato paste and sauce.	Regular canned vegetables and vegetable juices; regular tomato sauce and tomato paste; olives, sauerkraut, pickles; pickled vegetables; frozen vegetables in butter or sauces; vegetables seasoned with ham, bacon, or salt pork; processed potato preparations. Some frozen vegetables, like peas and lima beans are treated with salt.
Fruits	Most fresh, frozen, dried, and canned fruits.	Fruits processed with salt or sodium-containing salt as an ingredient (some dried fruits are processed with sodium sulfites); and picked fruits.
Low-fat dairy	Milk; eggnog; yogurt; low sodium ricotta or cottage cheese; cream cheese; low sodium cheese; and sour cream.	Malted milk; buttermilk, milkshakes; chocolate milk; cheese; and processed cheese and cheese spreads.
Meat/Beans	Any fresh or frozen beef, lamb, pork, poultry, fish, and shrimp; low sodium canned tuna or salmon, rinsed; eggs and egg substitutes; low-sodium peanut butter; dried peas and beans;	Any smoked, cured, salted, koshered, or canned meat, fish, or poultry including bacon, chipped beef, ham, hot dogs, and sausage. Sardines,

	eggs; frozen dinners (<500 mg sodium).	anchovies, crab, lobster, imitation seafood, marinated herring, and pickled meats; frozen breaded meats; regular canned tuna or salmon, luncheon meats, such as bologna and salami; pickled eggs; regular hard and processed cheese, cheese spreads and sauces; TV dinners, meat pies, and ***kosher meats*** *(see note below)*.
Beverages	All fruit juices, coffee, tea, low-sodium, salt-free vegetable juices, low-sodium carbonated beverages	Regular vegetable or tomato juices, carbonated diet beverages with sodium or salt added, commercially softened water used for drinking or cooking, for alcoholic beverages-check with a physician
Fats and Oils	Butter, margarine or mayonnaise; vegetable oils and shortenings; unsalted salad dressings, regular salad dressing limited to 1 Tbsp; light, sour, and heavy cream; salt-free gravies; and cream sauces.	Regular salad dressings containing bacon fat, bacon bits, bacon grease and salt pork; commercially prepared sauces and gravies; snack dips made with instant soup mixes or processed cheese; and salted nuts.
Soups	Low-sodium commercially canned and dehydrated soups, broths, and bouillons; homemade broth and soups without added salt and made with allowed vegetables; and cream soups.	Regular canned or dehydrated soups, broths, bouillon, and packaged and frozen soup.
Desserts and sweets	Gelatin, sherbet, fruit ices, fruits; pudding and ice cream as part of milk allowance; salt-free baked goods; sugar, honey, jam, jelly, marmalade and syrup	Instant pudding mixes and cake mixes; and chocolate candy
Condiments, sauces, miscellaneous	Salt substitute with physician's approval; pepper, herbs, allspice, caraway, cinnamon, cloves, curry powder, basil, bay leaf, marjoram, mustard powder, nutmeg, onion powder, fresh onion, oregano, paprika, poultry seasoning, garlic powder, fresh garlic, thyme, sage, rosemary; vinegar, lemon or lime juice; hot pepper sauce; garlic powder, onion powder, low sodium soy sauce (1 T); low sodium condiments (ketchup, chili sauce, mustard, vinegar, Tabasco sauce) in limited amounts (1 tsp), fresh ground horseradish; unsalted tortilla chips, pretzels, potato chips, popcorn, salsa (1/4 cup), extracts (*e.g.* almond, lemon, vanilla), baking chocolate and cocoa, and seasoning blends that do not contain salt, such as "Mrs. Dash."	Table salt, light salt, any seasoning made with salt including garlic salt, bouillon cubes, meat extract, celery salt, onion salt, and seasoned salt; sea salt, rock salt, kosher salt; meat tenderizers, meat extract; monosodium glutamate; mustard, regular soy sauce, tartar sauce, barbecue sauce, chili sauce, teriyaki sauce, steak sauce, Worcestershire sauce, and most flavored vinegars; canned gravy and mixes; regular condiments; salted snack foods, olives, pickles, relish, horseradish sauce, and ketchup.

Note on kosher meat: The salt content of kosher meats has not been well studied, but is likely to be higher than non-kosher meat. [21-22] Individuals on salt restricted diets should be advised of this and advised to buy commercially kashered meat, which may absorb less salt than home kashered meats.[23] Other ways to reduce sodium in the diet should also be discussed with observant Jews needing a salt restriction. Reduction of meat intake is one option, but reducing consumption of processed foods and increased use of herbs or lemon should also be explored. It is important to accommodate patient's cultural, ethnic, and religious preferences and requirements.

HELPFUL TIPS

- Snacking
    - Some good suggestions are:
        - Unsalted popcorn
        - Unsalted nuts
        - Crackers with unsalted tops with jelly or low sodium peanut butter
        - Fruit with low sodium cheese
        - Fresh vegetables and low sodium dip
- Food Preparation
    - Meats:
        - Pork: sage, onion; serve with applesauce
        - Chicken: poultry seasoning, thyme, parsley; serve with cranberry sauce
        - Lamb: curry powder, rosemary, garlic, thyme; serve with mint sauce/jelly
        - Veal: marjoram, basil; serve with currant jelly or cranberry sauce
        - Beef: pepper, bay leaf; serve with dry mustard, unsalted chive butter
    - Fish: bay leaf, dill: serve with unsalted lemon or parsley butter
    - Vegetables:
        - Asparagus: lemon juice
        - Broccoli: lemon juice
        - Carrots - mustard dressing, parsley, mint, dill, glazed with unsalted butter and sugar
        - Green beans: marjoram, lemon juice, nutmeg, dill seed
        - Tomatoes: basil, marjoram, onion

In situations where a sodium restriction less than 2,000 mg is needed (1,500 mg, 1,000 mg, or less) it may be necessary to purchase low sodium bread, low sodium milk, and to eschew most condiments. These foods are difficult to find and may be expensive. Most condiments should be eschewed. Frozen peas may also be treated with salt during processing and individuals should check the label of individual products. The sodium content of prescription and over the counter medications should be considered--patients should discuss this with their pharmacist. For residents/patients needing *more sodium* in their diet, for example, patients on lithium or patients on a liberalized geriatric menu, salt can be added at the table by the resident/patient or by an aide. Some individuals may find a low-sodium diet untenable; if approved by their physician, salt packets can be provided with meals and salt can be added at the table. In addition, herbs, spices, and lemon juice or vinegar can be used as desired. It may be helpful to determine actual intake of patients on low sodium diets--if they are not meeting their assessed energy needs, patients may not be approaching 2,000 mg of sodium and more salt may help increase intake.

REDUCED SODIUM DIET

Food Groups	Servings/Day	Allowed Foods	Foods to Avoid
Grains	6 ounces; 3 or more of which should be whole grains	Enriched white, wheat, rye, and other breads. Ready-to-eat cereals, cooked cereals, rolls, crackers without salted tops, low-sodium snack crackers, bread sticks, cooked grain products.	Salted crackers, chips and snack items; prepared breads, cornbread, biscuits (1 per day); regular bread limited to 3 servings per day; low sodium breads. Commercially available products such as macaroni and cheese or products cooked with spice mixes or broth. Packaged stuffing mixes or pre-mixed baking products.
Vegetables	2.5 cups	Fresh, frozen, or canned without sodium or drained and washed. Low sodium vegetable juices. No salt added vegetable soups.	Regular canned vegetables, baked beans, sauerkraut, regular canned vegetable juices. Frozen vegetables in sauces.
Fruit	2 cups	All fresh, frozen, canned, and 100% fruit juices	None
Milk/Dairy	3 cups	Fat-free or low-fat milk, yogurt, ice milk, or sherbet.	Buttermilk, malted milk, milk shakes.
Meat/Beans	5.5 ounces	All fresh or frozen beef, pork, veal, game, shellfish, fish, eggs, tuna; cheese in limited amounts or low-salt cheese; dried beans and peas; salt-reduced peanut butter.	Smoked, cured, salted, or regularly canned meats, processed meats, seafood, poultry, processed cheese, regular peanut butter, and cottage cheese. Commercially available TV dinners and meat pies.
Oils	6 teaspoons	Regular butter or margarine in limited amounts, salt-free margarine or butter, cream, non-dairy creamers, oil, sour cream whipped topping, low-sodium, mayonnaise, and salad dressings, salt-free gravy.	Cream cheese, regular mayonnaise or salad dressings, snack dips made with instant mixes, and salted fats. Bacon grease and salt pork.
Discretionary Calories	With 2,000 kcals, limit to 265 kcals	Coffee, tea, decaffeinated coffee, regular or diet carbonated beverages, unsalted baked products, diet gelatin. Plain cake and cookies, regular custard and pudding, ice cream, syrup, jam, jelly, hard candies, marshmallows, plain milk chocolate candy, spices, herbs, salt-free seasoning and extracts, Tabasco sauce, dry mustard, and low sodium ketchup.	Instant pudding mixes, candy bars, seasoned salts, pickles, pickled relishes, monosodium glutamate, and regular ketchup. Barbeque sauces, soy sauces, oyster sauces, are also high in sodium.

REDUCED SODIUM DIET				
Sample Menu Plan	**Sample Menu**	**Portions**	**Nutrient Content Food Groups**	
Breakfast			Energy (kcals)	2154
Grain	Whole Wheat Toast	1 slice	Protein (g [%])[2]	95.72 [17.8]
Grain	Oatmeal	½ cup	Carbohydrates (g [%])	309.98 [57.6]
Fruit	Banana	1 med	Total Lipid (g [%])	61.75 [25.8]
Fruit	Orange Juice	½ cup	SFA (g [%])	14.51 [6.1]
Dairy	Fat Free Milk	1 cup	MUFA (g [%])	26.40 [11.0]
Meat	Scrambled Egg Substitute	¼ c raw	PUFA (g [%])	16.25 [6.8]
Oil	Trans-Fat Free Margarine	1 t	Cholesterol (mg)3	111
Discretionary Kcals	Jelly	1 T	Fiber (g)	29.6
Beverage	Coffee	1 cup	Vitamin A (IU)	30815
Lunch			Vitamin E (mg)	7.09
Grain	Whole Wheat Bun	1 bun	Vitamin K (mcg)	97.5
Meat	Chicken Breast/canola oil	2 oz/2t	Vitamin C (mg)	102.5
Vegetable	Lettuce, Shredded	½ cup	Thiamin (mg)	2.237
Vegetable	Tomato	2 slices	Riboflavin (mg)	2.995
Other	Yellow mustard	2 t	Niacin (mg)	27.713
Vegetable	Baked Sweet Potato	½ cup	Pantothenic Acid (mg)	9.556
Vegetable	Corn	½ cup	Vitamin B6 (mg)	2.549
Fruit	Fruit Salad	1 cup	Folate (mcg)	424
Dairy	Fat Free Milk	1 cup	Vitamin B12 (mcg)	6.3
Oil	Trans-Fat Free Margarine	1 t	Sodium (mg)	1685
Beverage	Iced Tea, Unsweetened	1 cup	Potassium (mg)	4821
Dinner			Calcium (mg)	1460
Meat/Oil	Catfish, Baked in canola oil	2 ½ oz/2t	Iron (mg)	18.29
Grain	Brown Rice	½ cup	Magnesium (mg)	495
Grain	Dinner Roll	1 small	Phosphorus (mg)	1820
Vegetable	Black Eyed Peas	½ cup	Zinc (mg)	11.27
Vegetable	Mustard Greens	½ cup		
Fruit	Canned Pineapple	½ cup		
Oil	Trans-Fat Free Margarine	1 t		
Beverage	Iced Tea, Unsweetened	1 cup		
Snack				
Grain	Graham Crackers	3		
Fruit	Apple Sauce	½ cup		
Dairy	Fat Free Milk	1 cup		

DASH Diet

INTENDED USE

The Dietary Approaches to Stop Hypertension (DASH) Eating Plan is intended to lower blood pressure and treat Hypertension through the decreased consumption of sodium (<2400 mg/day) and increased consumption of potassium (4700 mg), magnesium (500 mg), calcium (1240 mg), and fiber (30 gm) within 2000 kcals and 90 grams of protein.[24-42]

ADEQUACY

This diet is adequate and meets the Dietary Reference Intakes (DRIs) as established by the Institite of Medicine's food and Nutrition Board (FNB) for adult makles and females. The sample menu here provides 2000 kcals per day and meets MyPlate recommendations for food groups.

GENERAL DESCRIPTION

The DASH diet based on 2,000 kcals contains the following number of servings of each food group:
- 7-8 servings of grains (3 whole grains)
- 4-5 servings of fruit
- 4-5 servings of vegetables
- 2-3 servings of low-fat or nonfat dairy products
- 2 or less servings of lean meat, fish or poultry
- 4-5 servings of nuts, seeds, legumes weekly
- Limited fats and sweets
- Limit sodium intake (see Reduced Sodium diet for tips)

Sample DASH Menu

Meal	2,000 calories and 2,300 mg Sodium Menu
Breaskfast	3/4 cup bran flakes cereal
	1 medium banana
	1 cup low-fat milk
	1 slice whole wheat bread
	1 tsp soft (tub) margarine
	1 cup orange juice
Lunch	3/4 cup chicken salad
	2 slices whole wheat bread
	1 Tbsp Dijon mustard

	Salad of 1/2 cup fresh cucumber slices, ½ cup tomato wedges, 1 Tbsp unsalted sunflower seeds, 1 tsp Italian dressing, low calorie
	1/2 cup fruit cocktail, juice pack
Dinner	3 oz beef, eye of the round
	2 Tbsp beef gravy, fat-free
	1 cup green beans, sautéed with
	1/2 tsp canola oil
	1 small baked potato
	1 Tbsp sour cream, fat-free
	1 Tbsp grated natural cheddar cheese, reduced fat
	1 Tbsp chopped scallions
	1 small whole wheat roll
	1 tsp soft (tub) margarine
	1 small apple
	1 cup low-fat milk
Snacks	1/3 cup almonds, unsalted
	1/4 cup raisins
	1/2 cup fruit yogurt, fat-free, no sugar added

*Menu adapted from The National Heart, Lung, and Blood Institute[43]

CARDIAC MANAGEMENT

INTENDED USE
This diet is used for the management of coronary artery disease, peripheral artery disease, stroke, and dyslipidemia. The diet is often coupled with a reduced sodium diet, since many patients have coronary artery disease and hypertension, congestive heart failure or renal disease.

ADEQUACY
This diet is adequate and meets the Dietary Reference Intakes (DRIs) as established by the IOM's FNB for male and female adults.

RECOMMENDATIONS
Following a dietary plan called Therapeutic Lifestyle Changes (TLC) can help people who have high amounts of cholesterol in their blood to achieve desirable blood lipid ranges. This plan follows the recommendations of the National Cholesterol Education Program Adult Treatment Panel III; similar recommendations are given by the American Heart Association. A Dietary Approaches to Stop Hypertension, a Mediterranean Diet, or a diet from the American Diabetes Association may also be appropriate for some cardiac patients. The Academy of Nutrition and Dietetics also has a position paper on dietary fatty acids.[1] Many people with heart disease should also follow an energy controlled diet. This diet should be individualized to meet the person's nutritional needs.[2] Small frequent feedings may be better tolerated than three large meals per day. Sufficient energy is needed for the person to achieve and maintain desirable body weight.

Nutrient Composition of the TLC Diet[3]

Nutrient	Recommended Intake
Saturated Fat	Less than 7% of total kcal
Polyunsaturated Fat	Up to 10% of total kcal
Monounsaturated Fat	Up to 20% of total kcal
Total Fat	25-35% of total kcal
Cholesterol	<200 mg/day
Carbohydrate	50-60% of total kcal
Fiber	20-30 g/day
Protein	~ 15% of total kcal
Sodium	<2400 mg/day
Stanol Esters	3-4 g/day

Source: U.S. Department of Health and Human Services, Public Health Service, National Institutes of Health, National Heart, Lung, and Blood Institute, NIH-Publication No. 01-3305; May 2001.

TLC Diet Recommendations[3]

Limit total fat intake to 25% to 35% of the calories. If you should eat 2,000 calories per day, your fat intake can be between 50 and 75 grams (g) per day.	Example:A person who consumes 2,000 calories a day should consume between 50-75 grams of fat per day.
Limit saturated fats and trans fats:	• Foods high in saturated fats include fatty meat, poultry skin, bacon, sausage, whole milk, cream, and butter. • Trans fats are found in stick margarine, shortening, some fried foods, and packaged foods made with hydrogenated or partially hydrogenated oils. Check the ingredient labels. • Replace butter or stick margarine, with reduced-fat, whipped, or liquid spreads.
Limit the amount of cholesterol consumed to less than 200 milligrams (mg) per day.	• Foods high in cholesterol include egg yolks, fatty meats, whole milk, cheese, and some seafood (shrimp, lobster, and crab).
Eat more omega-3 fats (heart-healthy fats):	• Good choices include salmon, tuna, mackerel, and sardines and these should be consumed twice a week. • Walnuts, flax seed, flax seed oil, canola and soybean oils are also good sources of omega-3 fats.
Get 20 to 30 g of dietary fiber per day:	Fruits, vegetables, whole grains, and dried beans are good sources of fiber. • Consume 5 servings of fruits and vegetables per day. • Consume 3 ounces of whole grain foods per day. • Eat more plant based meals which include legumes.

Potential long term adverse effects of alcohol preclude health care professionals from recommending alcohol consumption. If consumed, alcohol should be limited to two drinks per day for men and one drink per day for women. In some individuals who already drink alcohol, red wine may be associated with cardiac benefits. Individuals with high triglyceride levels should eschew from alcohol and simple sugars.[3]

The recommendations for SFA intake and trans-fat intake are rated by the Evidence Analysis Library of the Academy of Nutrition and Dietetics as "Strong, Imperative."[1]

CARDIAC DIET			
Food Groups	**Servings/Day**	**Allowed Foods**	**Foods to Limit**
Grains	6 ounces; 3 or more of which should be whole grains	Whole grain breads and cereal, enriched breads and cereal, pastas and rice, low fat or fat-free crackers, occasional use of biscuits, pancakes, muffins, French toast and waffles.	Granola or other high fat cereal, high fat chips, and crackers.
Vegetables	2.5 cups	Canned, frozen, and fresh from the following groups as recommended by the DGA and MyPlate: dark green, orange, starchy, dried peas and beans, and other	Those cooked in butter, cream sauce, cheese sauce or other high fat sauces. If patient has bloating and diarrhea: gaseous vegetables and dried beans may need to be avoided.
Fruit	2 cups	Canned, frozen, fresh, or dried fruits, and 100% fruit juices (no more than ⅓ of the requirement should be from 100% juice).	Coconut
Milk/Dairy	3 cups	Fat-free or low-fat milk, buttermilk, evaporated skim and nonfat dried milk, low fat or nonfat yogurt, and ice milk, and sherbet.	Whole milk dairy products including whole milk, whole flavored milks, yogurt, cheese, and ice cream.
Meat/Beans	5.5 ounces	Refer to the Diabetic Meat Exchange List. Use very-lean and lean meats including loin or round cuts of beef, pork, veal and lamb; poultry without skin; fish, shellfish, tuna canned in water; 95% fat free luncheon meats, egg white and egg substitutes, low fat cheeses; limit whole eggs to 7 per week.	Refer to Meat Exchange List. High fat varieties of beef, pork, lamb, luncheon meat, sausage, domestic duck and goose, fish canned in oil, poultry with skin, fried meats, excessive use of peanut butter (which is also high in salt).
Oils	6 teaspoons	Oils, soft, margarine, mayonnaise 1 tsp. = 1 serving Light margarine or mayonnaise, 1 Tbsp. = 1 serving Salad dressing, nuts, seeds 1 Tbsp. = 1 serving, bacon 1 slice = 1 serving	Fried foods and all fats in excess of 6 teaspoons per day.

Discretionary Calories	With 2,000 kcals, limit to 265 kcals	Jelly beans, gum drops, hard candies, suckers, pretzels, fat-free or low fat fruit bars, graham crackers, ginger snaps, animal crackers, vanilla wafers, angel food cake, Popsicles, gelatin, cocoa	All other cakes, cookies, pies, and pastries; puddings made with whole milk or eggs; cream puffs, large amounts of nuts, coconut and chocolate

2000 KCAL CARDIAC/DYSLIPIDEMIA DIET

Sample Plan	Sample Menu	Portion Size	Nutrient Analysis	
Breakfast			Energy (kcals)	2027
Grains	Whole Wheat Toast	1 slice	Protein (g [%])	96.41 [19.0]
	Oatmeal	½ cup	Carbohydrates (g [%])	313.6 [61.9]
Fruit	Banana	1 medium	Total Lipid (g [%])	48.41 [21.5]
	Orange Juice	½ cup	SFA (g [%])	12.63 [5.6]
Dairy	Fat-free Milk	1 cup	MUFA (g [%])	20.12 [8.9]
Meat Equivalent	Scrambled Egg Substitute	¼ cup raw	PUFA (g [%])	11.29 [5.0]
Oil	Soft Trans-Fatty Acid Free Margarine	1 t	Cholesterol (mg)	124
Discretionary	Jelly	1T	Fiber (g)	30.5
Beverage	Coffee	1 cup	Vitamin A (IU)	21469
Lunch			Vitamin E (mg)	19.7
Grains	Whole Wheat Bun	1 bun	Vitamin K (mcg)	735.9
Meat & Beans	Chicken Breast, No Skin Baked	2 oz	Vitamin C (mg)	184.6
Vegetables	Lettuce, Shredded	½ cup	Thiamin (mg)	3.28
Vegetables	Tomato	2 slices	Riboflavin (mg)	4.66
	Yellow Mustard	2 t	Niacin (mg)	45.34
Vegetables	Baked Sweet Potato "French Fries"	½ cup	Pantothenic Acid (mg)	18.98
Vegetables	Corn	½ cup	Vitamin B6 (mg)	4.62
Fruit	Fruit Salad	½ cup	Folate (mcg)	833
Dairy	Fat-free milk	1 cup	Vitamin B12 (mcg)	11.48
Oil	Margarine	2t	Sodium (mg)	2645
Oil	Canola oil	2t	Potassium (mg)	4710
Beverage	Iced Tea, Unsweetened	As desired	Calcium (mg)	1465
Dinner			Iron (mg)	33.06
Meat & Beans	Catfish	1 oz	Magnesium (mg)	506
Grains	Whole wheat dinner roll	1 roll	Phosphorus (mg)	1751
Grains	Brown rice	½ cup	Zinc (mg)	27.27
Fruit	Canned pineapple	½ cup		
Vegetables	Spinach	½ cup		
Vegetables	White beans[1]	½ beans		
Dairy	Fat free yogurt	1cup		
Oil	Canola Oil	2t		
Oil	Margarine	2t		
Beverage	Iced tea	As desired		
Bedtime Snack				
Fruit	Canned peaches	½ cup		

[1]The sodium in the diet can be reduced by washing canned beans under running water or using dried beans cooked without salt.

The diet above is consistent with the NCEP ATP III, AHA, Dietary Approaches to Stop Hypertension, and Dietary Guidelines for Americans recommendations for an adult requiring approximately 2,000 kcals/day. The diet is suitable for patients with coronary artery disease, stroke, hypertension, and diabetes.

Suggested Recipe Substitutions	
If Recipe Calls For:	Use This Instead:
Avocado	Asparagus or green peas pureed
Bacon	Canadian bacon
Bacon Bits	Soy bits Chicken or turkey without skin
Beef Bouillon Cubes	Low sodium broth or bouillon cubes
Butter	Equal amounts of apple sauce or other pureed fruit
Cheese	Fat-free cheese or lower fat versions
Chicken Stock	Vegetable stock or chicken stock with fat removed
Chocolate	3-4 Tbsp. Cocoa and 1 Tbsp. Canola oil
Chocolate Sauce	Fat-free chocolate syrup
Corn or Potato Chips	Baked low fat or no fat potato or corn chips
Cream	Non-fat dry milk or evaporated skim milk
Cream Cheese	Fat free or lower fat versions
Cream Sauce	Tomato sauce or cream sauce made with skim milk
Cream Soups	Prepare with non-fat dry milk or evaporated skim milk
Evaporated Milk	Evaporated skim milk
Flour and Oil Roux	No fat browned-flour roux
Fudge Sauce	Chocolate Syrup
Granola	Low fat granola or puffed cereal and raisins
Gravy	Butter flavored seasoning
Half and Half	Evaporated skim milk or Fat-Free half and half
Ice Cream	Fat-free or low fat ice cream
Icing	Powdered sugar or non-fat cream cheese blended with pineapple juice or skim milk Low fat or lower fat versions
Margarine	
Mayonnaise	Non-fat or lower fat versions
Oils in Baking	Applesauce, pureed prunes, pureed plums
Oils in Cooking, Frying, or Sautéing	Canola or olive oil Non-stock cookware or non-stick spray, water, non-fat broth, or wine
Peanut Butter	Reduced fat peanut butter or apple butter
Salad Dressing	Non-fat or lower fat versions
Salt/Seasoned Salts	Salt free herb blends
Shortening	For each cup required ¾ cup canola oil
Sour Cream	Low fat or non-fat sour cream or plain yogurt
Soy Sauce	Reduced sodium soy sauce
Wine	Non-alcoholic wine
Whipped Cream	Low fat/fat-free whipped cream substitute
White Flour	Whole wheat flour
White Pasta	Whole wheat pasta
White Rice	Brown rice
Whole Egg	Egg whites or ¼ cup egg substitute
Whole Milk	Fat-free or 1% low fat milk

DIETARY MANAGEMENT OF DIABETES

When recommending appropriate nutrition therapy, the dietitian may want to consider liberalizing standard diabetic diets for long-term care patients. Because regular institutional diets are at consistent meal times and are fairly consistent in nutrient composition, they may promote good glycemic control. Another benefit of a regular diet--without concentrated sweets, is the potential to improve quality of life, encourage intake, and promote weight gain if needed or weight loss or maintenance.

A dietitian's assessment should include: monthly weight, percent daily meal intake, fasting blood glucose, glycosylated hemoglobin levels, chewing and swallowing ability, ability to feed self, and activity level. Periodic assessment of glycemic control is important with this diet. An energy and carbohydrate-controlled meal plan can be used if control worsens.

According to the American Diabetes Association, there is no one best diet for individuals with diabetes. The ones presented here, include: regular, no concentrated sweets; the traditional exchange pattern, and diets planned on the glycemic index.

REGULAR, NO CONCENTRATED SWEETS

INTENDED USE This diet is intended for the individual with controlled type 2 diabetes mellitus who is at or near his desirable or goal weight as determined by the dietitian or physician. It may also be used for the person with Type 1 insulin dependent diabetes mellitus whose blood glucose and body weight are within acceptable ranges. Because of its varying carbohydrate content, the effects of this diet on blood sugar control should be monitored.

ADEQUACY The diet meets the Dietary Reference Intakes (DRIs) as established by the Institute of Medicine's Food and Nutrition Board (FNB) for adult males and females.

RECOMMENDATIONS
1. The regular diet should be used as the basis for this diet.
2. An effort should be made to distribute carbohydrate-rich foods evenly throughout the day.
3. Portion sizes on menu must be followed.
4. The meal plan consists of three meals and a bedtime snack unless indicated otherwise.
5. A sugar substitute may be used as a sweetening agent.
6. Dessert items such as cake, pudding, and regular gelatin desserts should be replaced with fresh fruit or fruit canned in juice (without sugar), sugar-free pudding, or sugar-free gelatin desserts. The Other Carbohydrates list can be used for increased variety.
7. Patients with diabetes are at high risk for heart disease, hypertension, and renal disease and should be monitored for signs and symptoms of these diseases and their diet may need to be modified accordingly.
8. Intake of saturated fatty acids (SFA) should be <7% of total energy and intake of trans-fat should be minimized.

Note on No-Concentrated Sweets Diet for patients in nursing homes: The literature confirming the suitability of this diet for the elderly, including the free-living elderly and those confined to long-term care facilities is sparse.[1] One small study compared nursing home patients (n=14) with type 2 diabetes mellitus consuming a no-concentrated sweets diet to those consuming a regular diet (n=14). At 3 and 6 months, there were no differences in mean glycated hemoglobin, mean fasting blood glucose, mean glucose, and albumin levels, or in body mass index between the two groups. These data are clearly limited; however it should be noted that in 1999 the American Diabetes Association recommended serving a regular diet to those patients in long term care to reduce the risk of malnutrition.[2] With such limited evidence, it is difficult to recommend that a no-concentrated sweets diet be used; however, one is presented herein--it is based on a regular diet and patient tolerance should be monitored. Hemoglobin A1c should be monitored at least twice yearly with a goal should be <7%.

Food Choices for Patients on No Concentrated Sweets Diets			
Foods to Choose	**Foods to Limit**	**Foods to Choose**	**Foods to Limit**
Grains: Unsweetened crackers such as Akmak, graham crackers, animal crackers, bread sticks, saltines, Zwieback, pretzels (soft and hard), Melba toast, and unsweetened rice cakes. Matzah, unsweetened whole grain breads, hamburger and hot-dog buns, English muffins, bagels, rolls, tortillas, and pita bread. Unsweetened Ready-to-eat cereals, cooked cereals, grits, and barley. Bulgur, pasta, rice, and couscous. Pancakes, waffles, muffins, and biscuits made with allowed ingredients.	*Grains:* Cinnamon, sweetened, or frosted breads. Any bread prepared with sweetened sauces. Sweet rolls, doughnuts, coffee cakes, pastries, Danish rolls, muffins and any with added honey or sugar. Pre-sweetened or granola-type cereals.	*Fats and Snacks:[1]* Margarine or butter. Sugar free gelatin desserts and custards. Angel food cake, vanilla wafers, gingersnaps, sugar-free cocoa mixes; air-popped popcorn.	*Fats and Snacks:* Frozen whipped toppings such as Cool Whip, Dream Whip, or Reddi Whip. Salad dressings with sugar as one of first three ingredients. Ice cream, sherbet, sorbet, fruit ice, Popsicles,[2] gelatin.[2] Frosted cakes, cupcakes, pie, puddings, pastries, candy, fruit rolls, caramelized popcorn, Pop-tarts,® granola bars, or breakfast bars.
Fruit: Fresh or frozen fruits processed without sugar	*Fruit:* Canned, fresh or frozen fruit with sugar or syrup		

Water-packed canned fruits 100% juices	Sweetened fruit flavored drinks, blended juices, nectars		
Vegetables: All fresh, canned, frozen or cooked vegetables. Peans, corns and potatoes.	*Vegetables:* Candied sauced or glazes cooked with honey, syrup, sugar, jelly, marmalade, or jam.		
Milk: Milk (whole [limit], skim, low fat, or buttermilk); plain low-fat yogurt (sweetened with fresh fruit or cinnamon); and cheese, all kinds.	*Milk:* Fruited or flavored yogurt; milkshake, frozen malt or frozen milkshake; Nestle's Quick powders, flavored milk; instant breakfast type drinks; sweetened cocoa mixes; chocolate milk; and eggnog.	*Miscellaneous:* Water, carbonated or mineral waters (sugar-free), club soda; sugar-free sodas; coffee, decaffeinated coffee; tea; or sugar-free mixers. Salt and soy sauce (if not on low sodium diet). Pepper, herbs, spices, garlic, meat sauce (*e.g.* Worcestershire sauce, A-1 sauce). Hot sauce, mustard, dill pickles, and olives.	*Miscellaneous:* Regular carbonated beverages or soft drinks; sweetened fruit drinks, Kool-Aid and Hi-C; tonic water, beer, wine, alcohol, and hard liquor; barbeque sauce, ketchup, teriyaki sauce, sugar, honey, fructose, molasses, and corn syrup. Sweet pickles, pickle relish, jelly, jam, or syrup. Regular chewing gum. Most prepared sauces.
Meat & Beans: Chicken, turkey, fish, beef, lamb, pork, veal; dried beans, peas, or lentils; peanut butter; eggs.	*Meat & Beans:* Any meat, poultry or fish prepared with sweet and sour marinades (made with sugar), barbecue sauces that have ketchup, chili sauce, honey or brown sugar, and teriyaki sauce. Baked beans flavored with brown sugar, molasses, honey or maple syrup.	*Label Ingredients:* All others.	*Label Ingredients:* Brown sugar, chocolate, corn syrup, corn syrup solids, dextrose, fructose, Glucose, high fructose corn syrup, honey, lactose, maltose, mannitol, modified food starch, molasses, natural sweeteners, sorbitol, sucrose, sugar, and syrups.

[1]Monounsaturated and polyunsaturated fats are preferred fats and oils.
[2]Sugar-free versions are available

NO CONCENTRATED SWEETS DIETS

Sample Menu Plan	Sample Menu	Portion Size	Nutrient Analysis	
Breakfast			Energy (kcals)	1954
Whole Grain	Whole Wheat Toast	1 slice	Protein (g [%])	92.19 [19]
Whole Grain	Oatmeal	½ cup	Carbohydrates (g [%])	264.14 [54]
Fruit	Banana	1 med	Total Lipid (g [%])	60.97 [28]
Dairy	Fat-Free Milk	1 cup	SFA (g [%])	14.36 [6.6]
Meat	Scrambled Egg Substitute	¼ c raw	MUFA (g [%])	26.22 [12]
Oil	Trans-Fat Free Margarine	1 t	PUFA (g [%])	15.93 [7.3]
Beverage	Coffee	1 cup	Cholesterol (mg)	111
Lunch			Fiber (g)	27.2
Whole Grain	Whole Wheat Bun	1 bun	Vitamin A (IU)	25064
Meat	Chicken Breast/canola oil	2 oz/2 t	Vitamin E (mg)	7.18
Vegetable	Lettuce, Shredded	½ c	Vitamin K (mcg)	146.3
Vegetable	Tomato	2 slices	Vitamin C (mg)	123.1
Other	Yellow Mustard	2 t	Thiamin (mg)	2.19
Vegetable	Baked Sweet Potato	½ cup	Riboflavin (mg)	2.88
Vegetable	Steamed Cabbage	½ cup	Niacin (mg)	25.69
Fruit	Fruit Salad	½ cup	Pantothenic Acid (mg)	9.37
Dairy	Fat-Free Milk	1 cup	Vitamin B6 (mg)	2.49
Oil	Trans-Fat Free Margarine	1 t	Folate (mcg)	324
Beverage	Iced Tea, Unsweetened	1 cup	Vitamin B12 (mcg)	6.3
Dinner			Sodium (mg)	1826
Meat/Oil	Catfish, Baked in canola oil	2½ oz/2 t	Potassium (mg)	4266
Whole Grain	Brown Rice	⅓ c	Calcium (mg)	1385
Refined Grain	Dinner Roll	1 small	Iron (mg)	17.32
Vegetable	Green Beans	½ cup	Magnesium (mg)	434
Vegetable	Carrots	½ cup	Phosphorus (mg)	1725
Fruit	Canned Pineapple in Juice	½ cup	Zinc (mg)	10.01
Oil	Trans-Fat Free Margarine	1 t		
Beverage	Iced Tea, Unsweetened	1 cup		
Snack				
Grain	Graham Crackers	3 crackers		
Fruit	Canned Pears	½ cup		
Dairy	Fat-Free Milk	1 cup		

DIABETIC, ENERGY CONTROLLED

INTENDED USE This diet is intended for the individual with controlled Type 1 and poorly controlled Type 2 diabetes mellitus or the individual whose weight exceeds the recommended level for height and age as determined by the dietitian or physician. This diet should maintain blood glucose levels within an acceptable range. Depending on the energy level selected, it can be used to reach and maintain desirable body weight. Due to the composition of this diet, it can also aid in improving blood lipids of the diabetic or obese individual and promote improvement in overall health through optimal nutrition.

ADEQUACY This diet meets the Dietary Reference Intakes (DRIs) as established by the Institute of Medicine's Food and Nutrition Board (FNB) for adult males and females. Energy restricted to below 1500 kilocalories do not meet the DRIs and is not recommended or can be used with appropriate vitamin and mineral supplementation. The new guidelines include:

> Carbohydrate: Based on assessment
> Protein: 10-20% of kilocalories
> Saturated Fatty Acids (SFA): <7% SFA

The patterns on the following pages may be used.

RECOMMENDATIONS
1. When planning the menu, use the food exchange lists specifying correct serving sizes. Refer to the following pages for information on the food exchange lists.
2. Serving sizes on the menu must be followed.
3. The meal plan consists of three meals and a bedtime snack unless specified otherwise.
4. A sugar substitute, approved by the dietitian, may be used as a sweetening agent. Many products, drinks and dietetic products use other sweeteners such as fructose, sorbitol, xylitol, or mannitol. These contain energy, and if used, must be calculated as part of the diet. Some simple sugar may be consumed, but it too must be calculated as part of the diet.
5. Suggested meal patterns for 1500, 1800, and 2000 calories are provided on the following pages. The calorie level requirement of a resident is based on the nutrition assessment performed by a Licensed Dietitian/Nutritionist.
6. In overweight individuals, weight loss should not exceed 1 to 2 pounds weekly.

SUGGESTED MEAL PATTERNS DIABETIC AND CALORIE-CONTROLLED DIETS

Food Groups	Energy Guides					
	1500 kcals		1800 kcals		2000 kcals	
Exchange	#	Foods	#	Foods	#	Foods
Breakfast						
Starch/Bread	2	2 slices WW toast	2	½ cup oatmeal, 1 slice WW toast	3	¾ cup cereal, 1 slice WW toast*
Meat	1	1 HB egg	1	1 scrambled egg	1	1 poached egg
Fruit	1	½ cup peaches	1	½ cup apple juice	1(2)	½ cup orange juice ½ cup strawberries
Milk, fat-free	1	1 cup	1	1 cup	1	1 cup
Fat	1	1 t margarine	1	1 t margarine	1	1 t margarine
Other		Coffee		Coffee		Coffee
Lunch						
Starch/Bread	2	Vegetable Soup/1 slice WW bread	3	2 slices WW bread†	3	½ cup mashed potatoes, 1 small rollΩ
Meat	1	1 ½ oz cheese	2	2 ounces ham	3	Pot roast
Vegetable	1-2	½ cup green beans	2	½ cup cabbage (slaw) ½ cup spinach	2	½ carrots ½ cup string beans
Fruit	1	½ cup pineapple	1	1 small banana	2	1 cup peaches
Fat	2	1 t mayonnaise 1 t margarine	2	2 t mayo + vinegar	2	Gravy ½ cupΩ
Other		Iced tea		1 cup milk†		½ cup milk Ω
Dinner						
Starch/Bread	2	½ cup mashed potatoes; 1 small roll	3	½ cup mashed potatoes; 1 small roll	3	2 slices WW bread
Meat	2	2 oz pot roast	2	2 oz pot roast	2	2 oz turkey
Vegetable	1-2	½ cup spinach ½ cup carrots	2	½ cup string beans‡ ½ cup carrots‡	2	½ cup beets ½ cup spinach
Fruit	1	1/2 cup applesauce	1	½ cup applesauce	1	½ medium banana
Milk, fat-free	1	1 cup	1	1 cup	1	1 cup milk
Fat	1	1 t margarine	2	Gravy	2	2 t mayonnaise
Other		Salad greens with 1 T fat free dressing				Salad greens
Bedtime Snack						
Starch	1	½ cup sugar-free pudding	1	3 graham crackers	1	3 graham crackers
Milk	--		1	1 cup fat-free milk	1	1 cup fat-free milk
CALORIES		1520		1825		2090
GM CHO		204 (52%)		224 (49%)		254 (50%)
GM PRO		71 (19%)		86 (19%)		96 (19%)
GM FAT		54 (31%)		64 (32%)		70 (30%)

*Substitute one carbohydrate for 1 fruit; †substitute 1 carbohydrate for one milk; ‡ ¼ cup carrots and green beans are free foods--combination ~ ⅓ carbohydrate, other ½ carbohydrate is in the gravy; Ω Carbohydrates divided into gravy and ½ cup milk

If meat/protein is omitted at the breakfast meal, add one ounce of meat to lunch or supper plan.

Lean and medium-fat meat choices are used daily with high fat meats allowed three times weekly. Meats are calculated as medium fat.

Starch, fruit, and milk may have similar carbohydrate values and may occasionally be substituted for each other at a meal. However, nutritional needs may be compromised if this is done on a regular basis.

Plans are subject to approval of the dietitian and the physician at each facility and are to be modified, as necessary, to meet individual needs.

Adjustment of energy intake may be necessary to help individuals maintain desirable body weight. An individual should receive at least the minimum number of servings from each food group.

Energy intake can be decreased/reduced in the desired amount (100, 200 kilocalories) by removing/adding a food combination indicated in the appropriate example. It is emphasized that the diet should always contain the number of recommended servings in the Regular Diet for each food group. If it appears that less than the recommended number of servings would be required to reduce a resident's daily kilocalories to the needed low level, contact the Registered Dietitian. The following should not be used for diabetic meal plans.

1. Example – Each combination contains 100 kilocalories:

Combination A:
　One serving starch
　One half serving fat-free milk

Combination B:
　One ounce meat
　One serving vegetable

Combination C
　One serving fruit
　One serving vegetable

2. Example – Each combination contains 200 calories:

Combination A:	**Combination B**:
One serving starch	One serving fat-free milk
One serving fat	One serving fat
One ounce meat	One serving Starch

EXCHANGE LISTS FOR MEAL PLANNING

Serving a variety of foods selected from the different food groups assures that all essential nutrients are present. A familiar guide for grouping foods is the *Exchange Lists for Meal Planning*, a publication of the American Diabetes Association, Inc. and the American Dietetic Association.[3] Foods are grouped and listed together because they are similiar in the amounts of carbohydrate, protein, fat and calories they contain. When served in the amounts given, all choices in each list are equal. A food may be traded for any other food within the same food group; however, care should be taken or nutrient inadequacies can result.

The Food Group Lists Are:

The Starch List:
Bread Cereals and Grains
Starchy Vegetables, including beans, peas and lentils
Crackers and Snacks
Starchy Foods Prepared with Fat

The Fruit List:
Fruit, 100% Fruit Juice

The Milk List:
Fat-free and Low-fat Milk
Reduced-Fat Milk
Whole Milk

Sweets, Desserts, and Other Carbohydrates List

The Non-Starchy Vegetable List

The Meat and Meat Substitute List:
Lean meat
Medium-fat meat
High-fat meat
Plant-based protein

The Fat List:
Monounsaturated Fats
Polyunsaturated Fats
Saturated Fats

Combination Foods List

> The Exchange Lists are the basis of a meal planning system designed by a committee of the American Diabetes Association, Inc. and the Academy of Nutrition and Dietetics. While designed primarily for people with diabetes, the Exchange Lists are based on principles of good nutrition that apply to everyone.

STARCH LIST

Each serving of starch contains approximately 15 grams of carbohydrates, 3 grams of protein, a trace of fat, and 80 calories. Starch foods prepared with fat are higher in kilocalories and fat content. These foods should be limited to occasional use only.

Exchange List Foods--Starch			
Bread	**Food**	**Serving Size**	**Notes**
	Bagel, large (about 4 oz)	¼ (1 oz)	
	Biscuit	2½ " across	1 starch + 1 fat
	Bread, reduced calorie	1slice (1½ oz)	
	Bread, white, whole wheat, rye	1slice	
	Chapatti	6" across	
	Cornbread	1¾" cube	1 starch + 1 fat
	English muffin	½ muffin	
	Hot dog or hamburger bun	½ bun	
	Naan	8" x 2"	
	Pancake	4" across, ¼" thick	
	Pita	6" across, ½	
	Roll, plain, small	1 (1 oz)	
	Stuffing, bread	⅓ cup	
	Taco shell	5" across, 1	1 starch + 1 fat
	Tortilla, corn	6" across, 1	1 starch + 1 fat
	Tortilla, flour	6" across, 1	
	Tortilla, flour	10" across, ⅓	
	Waffle	4" square	1 starch + 1 fat
Cereal & Grains:	Barley, cooked	⅓cup	
	Bran, dry		
	Oat	¼ cup	
	Wheat	½ cup	
	Bulgur, cooked	½ cup	
	Cereals		
	Bran	½ cup	
	Cooked oats/oatmeal	½ cup	
	Puffed wheat or rice	1½ cups	
	Shredded wheat, plain	½ cup	
	Unsweetened, ready-to-eat	¾ cup	
	Couscous	⅓ cup	
	Granola		
	Low-fat	¼ cup	
	Regular	¼ cup	
	Grits, cooked	½ cup	
	Kasha	½ cup	
	Millet, cooked	⅓ cup	
	Musli	¼ cup	
	Pasta, cooked	⅓ cup	
	Polenta, cooked	⅓ cup	
	Quinoa, cooked	⅓ cup	
	Rice, white or brown, cooked	⅓ cup	
	Tabbouleh (prepared)	½ cup	
	Wheat germ, dry	3 T	

	Wild rice, cooked	½ cup	
Starchy Vegetables:	Cassava	⅓ cup	
	Corn	½ cup	
	Corn, on the cob	½ cob (5 oz)	
	Hominy, canned	¾ cup	
	Mixed vegetables with corn, peas, or pasta	1cup	
	Parsnips	½ cup	
	Peas	½ cup	
	Plantain, ripe	⅓ cup	
	Potato, baked with skin	¼ large (3 oz)	
	Potato, boiled all kinds	½ cup	
	Potato, mashed with milk and fat	½ cup	
	Potato, oven baked "fries"	1cup (2 oz)	
	Pumpkin, canned, no sugar added	1 cup	
	Squash, winter	1 cup	
	Succotash	½ cup	
	Yam, sweet potato, plain	½ cup	
Crackers and Snacks:	Animal crackers	8 crackers	
	Crackers, round-butter type	6 crackers	1 starch+ 1 fat
	Crackers, saltine-type	6 crackers	
	Crackers, sandwich-style, cheese/peanut butter filling	3 crackers	1 starch + 1 fat
	Crackers, whole-wheat regular	2-5 (¾oz)	1 starch + 1 fat
	Crackers, whole-wheat lower fat/crispbreads	2-5 (¾oz)	
	Crackers, graham	3 crackers	
	Matzah	¾ oz	
	Melba toast, 2" x 4"	20 crackers	
	Oyster crackers	3 cups	
	Popcorn, with butter	3 cups	
	Popcorn, no fat added	3 cups	1 starch + 1 fat
	Popcorn, lower fat	3 cups	
	Pretzels	¾ oz	
	Rice cakes, 4" diameter	2 cakes	
	Snack chips, fat-free or baked	15-20 (¾ oz)	
	Snack chips, regular	9-13 (¾ oz)	1 starch + 1 fat
Beans, Peas, and Lentils	Baked beans	⅓ cup	
	Beans, cooked	½ cup	
	Lentils, cooked	½ cup	
	Peas, cooked	½ cup	
	Refried beans, canned	½ cup	

FRUIT LIST

Certain items of this list contain rich sources of Vitamin A, Vitamin C, and fiber. Each serving of fruit contains approximately 15 grams of carbohydrate and 60 kilocalories. Unless otherwise noted, the serving size for one Fruit Exchange is: ½ cup of canned or fresh fruit or unsweetened fruit juice; 1 small piece of fresh fruit (~4oz), or 2 T of dried fruit.

Fresh, Frozen, Unsweetened Canned Fruit, and 100% Fruit Juice with Serving Size			
Fruit	**Serving Size**	**Fruit**	**Serving Size**
Apple, unpeeled, small	1 apple (4 oz)	Papaya	1 cup or ½ fruit
Apples, dried	4 rings	Peach, medium, fresh	1 peach (6 oz)
Applesauce (unsweetened)	½ cup	Peaches, canned	½ cup
Apricots, fresh	4 apricots (5½ oz)	Pear, large, fresh	½ (4 oz)
Apricots, dried	8 halves	Pears, canned	½ cup
Apricots, canned	1/2 cup	Pineapple, fresh	¾ cup
Banana, extra small	1 banana (4 oz)	Pineapple, canned	½ cup
Blackberries (raw)	¾ cup	Plums, canned	½ cup
Blueberries (raw)	¾ cup	Plums, dried	3 dried plums
Cantaloupe	⅓ melon (1 cup)	Plums, small	(5 oz)
Cherries, sweet, fresh	12 cherries (3 oz)	Raspberries	1 cup
Cherries, sweet, canned	½ cup	Strawberries	1¼ c whole berries
Dates	3	Tangerines, small	2 (8 oz)
Dried fruit (blueberries, cherries, cranberries, mixed fruit, raisins)	2 T	Watermelon	1 slice or 1¼ cup cubes
Figs, fresh	1½ lg or 2 med (3½ oz)		
Figs, dried	1½	**100% Fruit Juice**	**Serving Size**
Fruit Cocktail	½ cup	Apple juice/cider	½ cup
Grapefruit, large	½ grapefruit (11 oz)	Fruit juice blends	⅓ cup
Grapefruit sections, canned	¾ cup	Grape juice	⅓ cup
Grapes, small	17 grapes (3 oz)	Grapefruit juice	½ cup
Honeydew Melon	1 slice or 1 cup cubes	Orange juice	½ cup
Kiwi	1 (3½ oz)	Pineapple juice	½ cup
Mandarin Oranges, canned	¾ cup	Prune juice	⅓ cup
Mango, small	½ fruit (5½ oz) or ½ cup		
Nectarine, small	1 (5 oz)		
Orange, small	1 (6 ½ oz)		

MILK LIST

Each serving of milk or milk products on this list contains about 12 grams of carbohydrate and 8 grams of protein. The amount of fat in milk is measured in percent (%) of butterfat. The energy varies with the choice of milk. Since diabetics are at high risk for developing coronary artery disease, fat-free or skim milk is recommended. Skim milk and low-fat milk (1%) have 0-3 fat grams, reduced fat milk has 5 fat grams, and whole milk has 8 fat grams, in an 8 ounce serving.

Milk and Yogurts		
Food	Serving Size	Counts as
Fat-free or low-fat milk (1%)		
Milk, buttermilk, acidophilus milk, Lactaid	1 cup	1 fat-free milk
Evaporated milk	½ cup	1 fat-free milk
Yogurt, plain or flavored with an artificial sweetener	⅔ cup	1 fat-free milk
Reduced-fat (2%)		
Milk, acidophilus milk, kefir, Lactaid	1 cup	1 reduced-fat milk
Yogurt, plain	⅔ cup	1 reduced-fat milk
Whole		
Milk, buttermilk, goat's milk	1 cup	1 whole milk
Evaporated milk	½ cup	1 whole milk
Yogurt, plain	1 cup	1 whole milk

Other Dairy and Dairy-Like Foods		
Food	Serving Size	Counts as
Chocolate milk, fat free	1 cup	1 fat-free milk + 1 carbohydrate
Chocolate milk, whole	1 cup	1 whole milk + 1 carbohydrate
Eggnog, whole milk*	½ cup	1 carbohydrate + 2 fats
Rice drink, flavored low-fat	1 cup	2 carbohydrates + 2 fats
Rice drink, plain, fat-free	1 cup	1 carbohydrate
Smoothies, flavored regular	1 cup	1 fat-free milk + 2½ carbohydrates
Soy Beverage, light	1 cup	1 carbohydrate + ½ fat
Soy Beverage, regular plain	1 cup	1 carbohydrate + 1 fat
Yogurt, and juice blends	1 cup	1 fat-free milk + 1 carbohydrate
Yogurt, low carbohydrate	⅔ cup	½ fat-free milk
Yogurt, with fruit, low fat	⅔ cup	1 fat-free milk + 1 carbohydrate
*Use a pasteurized commercial preparation or prepare with pasteurized eggs.		

SWEETS, DESSERTS, AND OTHER CARBOHYDRATES

Moderate amounts of some foods can be used in the diabetic meal plan, in spite of their sugar or fat content, as long as the individual maintains blood-glucose control. Food choices from this list can be substituted for a starch, fruit, or milk exchange. However, they do not contain as many important vitamins and minerals as the choices on the Starch, Fruit, or Milk List.

Beverages, Soda, and Energy/Sports Drinks		
Food	**Serving Size**	**Counts as**
Cranberry juice cocktail	½ cup	2 carbohydrates
Energy drink	1can(8.3oz)	2 carbohydrates
Fruit drink or lemonade	1cup	2 carbohydrates
Hot chocolate, regular	1envelope and 1c water	1 carbohydrate
Hot chocolate, sugar-free	1 envelope and 1c water	1 carbohydrate
Soft drink (soda), regular	1 can (12oz)	2½ carbohydrates
Sports drink	1 cup	1 carbohydrate
Brownies, Cake, Cookies, Gelatin, Pie, and Pudding		
Food	**Serving Size**	**Counts as**
Brownie, small, unfrosted	1¼ inch square (1oz)	1 carbohydrate + 1fat
Cake, angel food, unfrosted	1/12 of cake (2 oz)	2 carbohydrates
Cake, frosted	2-inch square (2 oz)	2 carbohydrates + 1fat
Cake, unfrosted	2-inch square (2 oz)	1 carbohydrate + 1fat
Cookies, chocolate chip	2 cookies (2 ¼" across)	1 carbohydrate +2 fats
Cookies, gingersnaps	3 cookies	1 carbohydrate
Cookies, sandwich with cream filling	2 small (⅔ oz)	1 carbohydrate + 1 fat
Cookies, sugar free	3 small or 1 large (¾-1oz)	1 carbohydrate + 1-2 fats
Cookies, vanilla wafers	5 cookies	1 carbohydrate + 1fat
Cupcake, frosted	1 small (1¾oz)	2 carbohydrates + 1-1½ fats
Fruit cobbler	½ cup	3 carbohydrates + 1 fat
Gelatin, regular	½ cup	1 carbohydrate
Pie, commercial fruit, 2 crust	1/6 of 8" pie	3 carbohydrates + 2 fats
Pie, pumpkin or custard	⅛ of 8" pie	1½ carbohydrates + 1½ fats
Pudding, regular with 1% milk	½ cup	2 carbohydrates
Pudding, sugar free with skim milk	½ cup	1 carbohydrate
Candy, Spreads, Sweets, Sweeteners, Syrups, and Toppings		
Food	**Serving Size**	**Count as**
Candy bar, chocolate/peanut	2" (fun size) bars (1oz)	1 ½ carbohydrates + 1 ½ fats
Candy, hard	3 pieces	1 carbohydrate
Chocolate kisses	5 pieces	1 carbohydrate + 1 fat
Coffee creamer, dry flavored	4 t	½ carbohydrate + ½ fat
Coffee creamer, liquid flavored	2 T	1 carbohydrate
Fruit snacks, chewy	1 roll (¾ oz)	1 carbohydrate
Fruit spreads, 100% fruit	1½ T	1 carbohydrate
Honey	1 T	1 carbohydrate
Jelly or Jam, regular	1 T	1 carbohydrate
Sugar	1 T	1 carbohydrate

Syrup, chocolate	2 T	2 carbohydrates
Syrup, light (pancake)	2 T	1 carbohydrate
Syrup, regular (pancake)	1 T	1 carbohydrate

Condiments and Sauces

Food	Serving Size	Count as
Barbeque sauce	3 T	1 carbohydrate
Cranberry sauce, jellied	¼ cup	1 ½ carbohydrates
Gravy, canned or bottled*	½ cup	½ carbohydrate + ½ fat
Salad dressing, fat-free, low-fat, cream based	3 T	1 carbohydrate
Sweet and sour sauce	3 T	1 carbohydrate

Doughnuts, Muffins, Pastries, and Sweet Breads

Food	Serving Size	Count as
Banana Nut Bread	1 inch slice (1 oz)	2 carbohydrates + 1 fat
Doughnut, cake plain	1 medium (1½ oz)	1½ carbohydrates + 2 fats
Doughnut, yeast glazed	3¾" across (2 oz)	2 carbohydrates + 2 fats
Muffin (4 oz)	¼ muffin (1 oz)	1 carbohydrate + ½ fat
Sweet roll or Danish	1 (2½ oz)	2 ½ carbohydrates + 2 fats

Frozen Bars, Frozen Desserts, Frozen Yogurt, and Ice Cream

Food	Serving Size	Count as
Frozen pops	1 bar	½ carbohydrate
Fruit juice bars, frozen, 100% juice	1 bar (3 oz)	1 carbohydrate
Ice cream, fat-free	½ cup	1½ carbohydrates
Ice cream, light	½ cup	1 carbohydrate + 1 fat
Ice cream, no sugar added	½ cup	1 carbohydrate + 1 fat
Ice cream, regular	½ cup	1 carbohydrate + 2 fats
Sherbet, sorbet	½ cup	2 carbohydrates
Yogurt, frozen, fat-free	⅓ cup	1 carbohydrate
Yogurt, frozen, regular	½ cup	1 carbohydrate + 0-1 fat

Granola Bars, Meal Replacement Bars/Shakes, and Trail Mix

Food	Serving Size	Count as
Granola or snack bar	1 bar (1 oz)	1½ carbohydrate
Meal replacement bar	1 bar (1⅓ oz)	1 ½ carbohydrate + 0-1 fat
Meal replacement bar	1 bar (2 oz)	2 carbohydrates + 1 fat
Meal replacement shake	1 can (10-11 oz)	1½ carbohydrate + 0-1 fat
Trail mix, candy/nut-based	1 oz	1 carbohydrate + 2 fats
Trail mix, dried fruit-based	1 oz	1 carbohydrate + 1 fat

*480 mg or more of sodium

NON-STARCHY VEGETABLE LIST

Certain members of this list contain rich sources of Vitamin A, Vitamin C, and fiber. A food high in Vitamin A should be included in the diet at least every other day, and a food high in Vitamin C should be included daily.

Foods on the Vegetable list have approximately 5 grams of carbohydrate, 2 grams of protein and 25 kilocalories per ½ cup cooked or 1 cup raw serving. However, calories are increased if fat is used for seasoning. Vegetables contain 2-3 grams of dietary fiber.

Unless otherwise noted, the serving size for vegetables (one Vegetable Exchange) is: ½ cup of cooked vegetable or vegetable juice, 1 cup of raw vegetables. Vegetables containing 400 mg or more of sodium are identified with an (*).

Non-Starchy Vegetables	
Artichoke (½ medium)	Kohlrabi
Artichoke hearts	Leeks
Asparagus	Mixed vegetables (without corn, peas, or pasta)
Baby corn	Mung bean sprouts
Bamboo shoots	Mushrooms
Beans (Green, Wax, Italian)	Okra
Bean Sprouts	Onions
Beets	Pea Pods
*Borscht (soup)	Peppers (All varieties)
Broccoli	Radishes
Brussels Sprouts	Rutabaga
Cabbage (Green, bok choy, Chinese)	*Sauerkraut
Carrots	Soybean Sprouts
Cauliflower	Spinach
Celery	Sugar pea snaps
Chayote	Summer Squash (Summer, Crookneck, Zucchini)
Coleslaw (no dressing)	Swiss chard
Cucumber	Tomato
Daikon	Tomato, canned
Eggplant	*Tomato, sauce
Gourds (bitter, bottle, luffa, bitter melon)	*Tomato/Vegetable Juice
Green onions	Turnips
Greens (Collard, Mustard, Turnip)	Water Chestnuts
Hearts of palm	Zucchini, Cooked
Jicama	

MEAT LIST

Each serving of meat and substitutes on this list contains 7 grams of protein. Meats/meat substitutes that have 400 milligrams or more of sodium per exchange are indicated by an asterisk (*). The amount of fat and calories varies according to the type of meat/substitute chosen. The Meat Group is divided into four categories based on the amount of fat and energy. The four groups include lean meat, medium-fat meat, and high-fat meat. Most meat choices should be selected from the Lean Meat Category or from the plant-based protein group.

	Carbohydrates (g)	Protein (g)	Fat (g)	Energy (kcals)
Lean Meat	--	7	0-3	45
Medium-fat Meat	--	7	4-7	75
High-fat Meat	--	7	8+	100
Plant-based Protein	Varies	7	Varies	varies

Lean Meats and Meat Substitutes	
Food	**Amount**
Beef: Select of Choice grades trimmed of fat: ground round, roast (chuck, rib, rump), round, sirloin, steak (cubed, flank, porterhouse, T-bone), tenderloin	1 oz
*Beef Jerky	1 oz
Cheeses with 3 grams of fat or less/oz	1 oz
Cottage cheese	¼ cup
Egg substitutes, plain	¼ cup
Egg whites	2
Fish, fresh or frozen, plain: catfish, cod, flounder, haddock, halibut, orange roughy, salmon, tilapia, trout, tuna	1 oz
*Fish, smoked: herring or salmon	1 oz
Game: buffalo, ostrich, rabbit, venison	1 oz
†Hot dog with 3 grams of fat or less/oz (8 hot dogs/14 oz package)	1 oz
Lamb: chop, leg, roast	1 oz
‡Organ meats: heart, kidney, liver	1 oz
Oysters, fresh or frozen	6 medium
*Pork, lean, Canadian bacon	1 oz
Pork, lean, rib or loin chop/roast, ham, tenderloin	1 oz
Poultry, without skin: Cornish hen, chicken, domestic duck or goose (well-drained of fat), turkey	1 oz
Ω Processed sandwich meats with 3 g of fat or less/oz: chipped beef, deli thin-sliced meats, turkey ham, turkey kielbasa, turkey pastrami	1 oz
Salmon, canned	1 oz
Sardines, canned	2 medium
*Sausage with 3 g of fat or less/oz	1 oz
Shellfish: clams, crab, imitation shellfish, lobster, scallops, shrimp	1 oz
Tuna, canned in water or oil, drained	1 oz
Veal, lean chop, roast	1 oz
*480 mg or more of sodium; † May be high in carbohydrate; ‡ May be high in cholesterol; Ω May be high in sodium	

Medium-Fat Meats and Meat Substitutes

Food	Amount
Beef: corned, ground, meatloaf. Prime grades trimmed of fat (prime rib), short ribs, tongue	1 oz
Cheeses with 4-7 grams of fat/oz: feta, mozzarella, pasteurized processed cheese spread, reduced-fat cheeses, string	1 oz
‡Egg (limit to 3/week)	1 egg
Fish, any fried product	1 oz
Lamb: ground, rib roast	1 oz
Pork: cutlet, shoulder roast	1 oz
Poultry: chicken with skin, dove, pheasant, wild duck or goose, fried chicken, ground turkey	1 oz
Ricotta cheese	2 oz or ¼ cup
*Sausage with 4-7 g of fat/oz	1 oz
Veal, cutlet (no breading)	1 oz
*480 mg or more of sodium; ‡ May be high in cholesterol	

High-Fat Meats and Meat Substitutes

Food	Amount
*Bacon, pork	2 slices (2oz)
*Bacon, turkey	3 slices (1½ oz)
Cheese, regular: American, blue, brie, cheddar, hard goat, Monterey jack, queso, and Swiss	1 oz
*Δ Hot dog: beef, pork, or combination (10/lb package)	1
*Hot dog: turkey or chicken (10/lb package)	1
Pork: ground, sausage, spareribs	1 oz
Processed sandwich meats with 8 grams of fat or more/oz: bologna, pastrami, hard salami	1 oz
*Sausage with 8 grams of fat or more/oz: bratwurst, chorizo, Italian, knockwurst, Polish, smoked, summer	1 oz
*480 mg or more of sodium; Δ extra fat or prepared with added fat (add an additional fat choice to this food); ‡ May be high in cholesterol	

Plant-Based Proteins

Food	Amount	Counts as
"Bacon" strips, soy-based	3 strips	1 medium-fat meat
Baked beans	⅓ cup	1 starch + 1 lean meat
Beans, cooked: black, garbanzo, kidney, lima, navy, pinto, white	½ cup	1 starch + 1 lean meat
"Beef" or "sausage" crumbles, soy-based	2 oz	½ carbohydrate + 1 lean meat
"Chicken" nuggets, soy-based	2 nuggets	½ carbohydrate + 1 medium-fat meat
Edamame	½ cup	½ carbohydrate + 1 lean meat
Falafel	3 patties	1 carbohydrate + 1 high-fat meat
Hot dog, soy-based	1 (1½ oz)	½ carbohydrate + 1 lean meat
Hummus	⅓ cup	1 carbohydrate + 1 high-fat meat
Lentils, brown, green, or yellow	½ cup	1 carbohydrate + 1 lean meat
Meatless burger, soy-based	3 oz	½ carbohydrate + 2 lean meats

Meatless burger, vegetable- and starch-based	1 patty (2 ½ oz)	1 carbohydrate + 2 lean meats
Nut spreads: almond, cashew, or peanut butter, soy nut butter	1 T	1 high-fat meat
Peas, cooked: black-eyed and split peas	½ cup	1 starch + 1 lean meat
*Refried beans, canned	½ cup	1 starch + 1 lean meat
"Sausage" patties, soy-based	1 (1 ½ oz)	1 medium-fat meat
Soy nuts, unsalted	¾ oz	½ carbohydrate + 1 medium-fat meat
Tempeh	¼ cup	1 medium-fat meat
Tofu	½ cup	1 medium-fat meat
Tofu, light	½ cup	1 lean meat
*480 mg or more of sodium/serving		

FAT LIST

Fats are high in energy and should be measured carefully. Since saturated fatty acids (SFA) increase serum cholesterol levels, food sources of mono- and polyunsaturated fatty acids should be served more frequently than those with SFA. Each serving of fat contains approximately 5 grams of fat and 45 kilocalories.

Monounsaturated fatty acids	
Food	**Serving Size**
Avocado, medium	2 T
Nut butters (trans-fatty acid free): almond butter, cashew butter, peanut butter	1 ½ t
Tree Nuts and Peanuts:	
Almonds	6 nuts
Brazil	2 nuts
Cashews	6 nuts
Filberts	5 nuts
Macadamia	3 nuts
Mixed (50% peanuts)	6 nuts
Peanuts	10 nuts
Pecans	4 halves
Pistachios	16 nuts
Oil: canola, olive, peanut	1 t
Olives	
Black	8 large
Green, stuffed	10 large
Polyunsaturated fatty acids	
Food	**Serving Size**
Margarine: lower-fat spread (30-50% vegetable oil, trans-fatty acid free)	1 T
Margarine: stick, tub (trans-fatty acid free), or squeeze (trans-fatty acid free)	1 t
Mayonnaise	
Reduced-fat	1 T
Regular	1 t
Mayonnaise-style salad dressing	
Reduced-fat	1 T
Regular	1 t

Nuts	
Pine nuts	1 T
Walnuts, English	4 halves
Oil: corn, cottonseed, flaxseed, grape seed, safflower, soybean, sunflower	1 t
Oil: made from soybean and canola oil (Enova)	1 t
Plant stanol esters	
Light	1 T
Regular	2 t
*Salad dressings	
Reduced-fat (may be high in carbohydrates)	2 T
Regular	1 T
Seeds	
Flaxseed, whole	1 T
Pumpkin, sunflower	1 T
Sesame Seeds	1 T
Tahini	2 t

Saturated fatty acids	
Food	**Serving Size**
Bacon, cooked, regular or turkey	1 slice
Butter	
Reduced fat	1 T
Stick	1 t
Whipped	2 t
Butter blends made with oil	
Reduced-fat or light	1 T
Regular	1 ½ t
Chitterlings, boiled	2 T
Coconut, sweetened, shredded	2 T
Coconut milk	
Light	⅓ cup
Regular	1 ½ T
Cream	
Half and half	2 T
Heavy	1 T
Light	1½ T
Whipped	2 T
Whipped, pressurized	¼ cup
Cream cheese	
Reduced-fat	1½ T
Regular	1 T
Lard	1 t
Oil: coconut, palm, palm kernel	1 t
Salt pork	¼ oz
Shortening, solid	1 t
Sour cream	
Reduced-fat or light	3 T
Regular	2 T
*480 mg or more of sodium	

FREE FOODS: A free food is any food or drink that contains less than 20 calories per serving or less than 5 grams of carbohydrates per serving. Foods with a serving size listed should be limited to 3 servings per day. Spread them throughout the day to avoid affecting blood glucose levels. Foods listed without a serving size can be eaten freely.

Free Foods For Diabetics			
Low Carbohydrate Foods		*Modified Fat Foods With Carbohydrates*	
Cabbage, raw	½ cup	Cream cheese, fat-free	1 T
Candy, hard (regular or sugar free)	1 piece	Nondairy, liquid creamer	1T
Carrots, cauliflower, or green beans cooked	¼ cup	Nondairy, powdered creamer	2t
Cranberries, sweetened with sugar substitute	½ cup	Margarine spread, fat free	1 T
Cucumber, sliced	½ cup	Margarine spread, reduced-fat	1t
Gelatin, sugar free or unsweetened†		Mayonnaise, fat free	1T
Gum		Mayonnaise, reduced fat	1t
Jam or Jelly, light or no sugar added	2t	Salad dressing, fat-free or low-fat*	1T
Rhubarb, sweetened with sugar substitute	½ cup	Salad dressing, fat-free Italian*	2T
Salad greens		Sour cream, fat-free or reduced-fat	1T
Sugar substitutes		Whipped topping, light of fat-free	2T
Syrup, sugar free	2T	Whipped topping, regular	1T
†Foods without a serving size may be consumed with impunity; *May be high in sodium; check food label.			
Condiments		*Drinks/Mixes*	
Barbeque sauce	2t	Bouillon, broth, consommé*	
Ketchup	1T	Bouillon or broth, low-sodium	
Honey mustard	1T	Carbonated or mineral water	
Horseradish†		Club soda	
Lemon Juice		Cocoa powder, unsweetened	1T
Miso	1½ t	Coffee, unsweetened or with sugar sub	
Mustard		Diet soft drinks, sugar-free	
Parmesan cheese, freshly grated	1T	Drink mixes, sugar-free	
Pickle relish	1T	Tea, unsweetened or with sugar sub	
Pickles, dill*	1½ med	Tonic water, diet	
Pickles, bread and butter*	2 slices	Water	
Pickles, sweet gherkin	¾ oz	Water, flavored, carbohydrate free	
Salsa	¼ cup	*Seasonings*	
Soy sauce, light or regular*	1 T	Flavoring extracts, garlic, fresh or dried herbs, nonstick cooking spray, pimento, spices, hot pepper sauce, wine (in cooking), and Worcestershire sauce can all be used. However, seasons with "salt" in the name should be used with discretion--celery salt, onion salt, garlic salt. Try celery seeds, onion powder or onion, garlic powder or garlic.	
Sweet and sour sauce	2t		
Sweet chili sauce	2t		
Taco sauce	1T		
Vinegar			
Yogurt, any type	2 T		
†Foods without a serving size may be consumed with impunity; *High in sodium; check food label.			

Combination Foods		
Food	**Serving Size**	**Counts as**
*Casseroles (tuna noodle, lasagna, spaghetti and meatballs, chili with beans, macaroni and cheese)	1 cup	2 carbohydrates + 2 medium fat meats
*Stews (beef/other meats and vegetables)	1 cup	1 carbohydrate + 1 medium fat meat + 0/3 fats
Tuna or chicken salad	½ cup	½ carbohydrate + 2 lean meats + 1 fat
*Burrito (beef and bean)	1 (5 oz)	3 carbohydrates + 1 lean meat + 2 fats
*Dinner-type meal	14-17 oz	3 carbohydrates + 3 medium fat meats + 3 fats
*Entrée or meal with <340 kcals	~ 8-11 oz	2-3 carbohydrates + 1-2 lean meats
Pizza 　* Cheese/vegetarian 　*Meat topping, thin crust	¼ of 12" pie ¼ of 12" pie	2 carbohydrates + 2 medium fat meats 2 carbohydrates + 2 medium fat meats + 1-2 fats
*Pocket sandwich	1 (4 ½ oz)	3 carbohydrates + 1 lean meat + 1-2 fats
*Pot pie	1 (7 oz)	2 ½ carbohydrates + 1 medium fat meat + 3 fats
Salads		
Coleslaw	½ cup	1 carbohydrate + 1½ fats
Macaroni/pasta salad	½ cup	2 carbohydrates + 3 fats
*Potato salad	½ cup	1½ -2 carbohydrates + 1-2 fats
Soups		
*Bean, lentil, or split pea	1 cup	1 carbohydrate + 1 lean meat
*Chowder (made with milk)	1 cup	1 carbohydrate + 1 lean meat + 1½ fats
*Cream soup (made with water)	1 cup	1 carbohydrate + 1 fat
*Instant soup *Instant soup with beans or lentils	6 oz 8 oz	1 carbohydrate 2 ½ carbohydrates + 1 lean meat
*Miso soup	1 cup	½ carbohydrate + 1 fat
*Oriental noodle soup	1 cup	2 carbohydrates + 2 fats
Rice (congee)	1 cup	1 carbohydrate
*Tomato (made with water)	1 cup	1 carbohydrate
*Vegetable beef, chicken noodle, or other broth-type soups	1 cup	1 carbohydrate
*600 mg or more of sodium per serving = prepared foods; home-made foods will have less sodium		

MEAL PATTERN SUBSTITUTIONS FOR DIABETICS

Not every person on a diabetic or calorie-controlled diet will enjoy the exact menu pattern planned for the various calorie levels. Starch, fruit, and milk have similar carbohydrate values and may safely be substituted for each other at a given meal; however, nutritional needs may be compromised if this is done regularly.

To individualize the diet for these people, the menu patterns may be modified by making the following substitutions:

1. STARCH EXCHANGES:
   a. When one Starch/Carbohydrate Exchange is admitted: Add 1 Fruit Exchange or 1 Milk Exchange or 3 Non-Starchy Vegetable Exchanges

   b. When one Starch Exchange is added: Omit 1 Fruit Exchange or 1 Milk Exchange or 3 Non-Starchy Vegetable Exchanges

2. FRUIT EXCHANGES:

   a. When one Fruit Exchange is omitted: Add 1 Starch Exchange or 1 Milk Exchange or 3 Non-Starchy Vegetable Exchanges

   b. To add one Fruit Exchange: Omit 1 Bread Exchange or 1 Milk Exchange or 3 Non-Starchy Vegetable Exchanges

3. MILK EXCHANGES:

   a. When one Fat-free Milk Exchange is omitted: Add one Fruit or Starch Exchange and one Lean Meat Exchange

   b. To add one Fat-free Milk Exchange: Omit one Fruit or Starch Exchange and one Lean Meat Exchange

4. VEGETABLE EXCHANGES:

   Vegetable Exchanges are low in carbohydrates and calories and can be added or deleted by 1-2 exchanges.

Additional Resources: The National Institute of Diabetes, Digestive, and Kidney Diseases (NIDDK) have several resources for dietitians including the National Diabetes Education Program, which includes resources such as the **Guiding Principles for Diabetes Care.** The NIDDK also has a searchable database for publications on diabetes. To learn more about diabetes, the **Evidence Analysis Library** of the Academy of Nutrition and Dietetics has toolkits and on line resources.

GASTROINTESTINAL DIETS

LIBERAL BLAND DIET

INTENDED USE
The Liberal Bland Diet is commonly used as one of the modes of treatment for gastric ulcers, gastritis, or other gastrointestinal disorders. This diet includes restricting certain foods like caffeine, pepper, chocolate, and citrus juices that can irritate the Gastrointestinal (GI) tract and cause GI disturbances such as abdominal pain, bloating, heartburn, and diarrhea. *A diet should be individualized to accommodate each individual's intolerances.* Of common irritants, only alcohol has been shown to consistently irritate the gastrointestinal tract.

The National Institute of Diabetes, Digestive, and Kidney Diseases (NIDDK) does not have specific foods to be avoided for indigestion, but recommends eating several small, low-fat meals throughout the day at a slow pace and abstaining from consuming coffee, carbonated beverages, and alcohol. The NIDDK does not have any food or diet recommendations for peptic ulcer. For heartburn, Reflux Disease (GERD), the NIDDK recommends the avoidance of foods and beverages that worsen symptoms, east small, frequent meals, wear loose-fitting clothes, avoid lying down for 3 hours after a meal, and raise the head of the bed 6 to 8 inches by securing wood blocks under the bedposts.

For simple diarrhea, fluid replacement may be the only treatment necessary until the symptoms subside; caffeine, milk products, greasy foods, high in fiber, or very sweet should be avoided since these foods tend to aggravate diarrhea. Limiting foods and drinks that contain sugar (lactose, fructose, HFCS, corn syrup) and sugar alcohols (sorbital) is recommended, as well as eating small frequent meals and avoiding any food s that make diarrhea worse.[1] Patients with lactose maldigestion/malabsorption can generally tolerate some milk, although cheese and yogurt may be better tolerated. If they cannot tolerate milk, lactose reduced milk or lactase can be taken prior to consuming milk.[2]

ADEQUACY
Depending on individual tolerances, this diet may not meet the Dietary Reference Intakes (DRIs) as established by the Institute of Medicine's Food and Nutrition Board (FNB) for adult males and females for dietary fiber, vitamins C, D, E, and calcium since patients may be unable to consume fiber, citrus fruits, nuts/oils, or milk. If symptoms or adherence to the diet is prolonged, consider supplementation.

RECOMMENDATIONS

1. Interview the individual or family soon after admission or soon after the diet is ordered to determine individual tolerances/intolerances.
2. Recommend individual keeps an intolerance diary stating types and amount of foods consumed, time consumed, GI symptoms, and onset of symptoms to determine individual

food intolerances. Studies have shown that symptoms that start between 5-30 minutes after food consumption results from food intolerance.

3. Plan a nutritionally balanced diet for the individual, eliminating foods that appear to cause repeated GI disturbances.

4. Alcohol consumption is not advisable.

5. Vitamin and mineral supplement may be needed due to individual intolerances. For example, an individual who cannot tolerate acidic fruits and fruit juices may be deficient in Vitamin C. An individual who cannot tolerate milk or dairy products may be deficient in calcium, phosphorus, or riboflavin.

6. If the patient is given a bedtime snack to increase energy intake and experiences discomfort during the night, the nighttime snack should be omitted. Snacks should then be given throughout the day.

Foods Normally Tolerated on Liberal Bland Diets	
Grains	Plain white, rye or wheat bread; refined, cooked cereals such as cream of wheat, cream of rice, farina, strained oatmeal, puffed rice or wheat, cornflakes, crisp waffles; spaghetti, rice, noodles, macaroni; saltines, graham or plain crackers
Vegetables	Potatoes (mashed, baked or boiled), cooked asparagus tips, beets, carrots, green beans, mushrooms, pumpkin, winter squash, and sweet potatoes. Other vegetables may be tolerated by individuals.
Fruit	Stewed peaches, pears, apricots or baked apple without skins; canned peaches, pears, Royal Anne cherries, peeled apricots; applesauce, ripe banana, pureed fruits; ripe avocados; and all fruit juices except citrus juices.
Dairy	Whole, fat reduced, and skim milk; instant nonfat milk, evaporated milk, instant malted milk, instant breakfast, half and half, and buttermilk. Plain, mild-flavored cheeses (*e.g.,* American, cottage cheese)
Meats and Alternates	Broiled, boiled or roasted; ground or tender beef, veal, lamb, fresh pork, liver, chicken, turkey; baked, boiled or steamed fish such as cod, flounder, haddock, halibut and perch. Eggs Poached, scrambled, soft or hard boiled, baked, creamed; plain omelet or soufflé. Tofu or peanut butter. Crisp bacon.
Fats/oils	Butter, margarine, mayonnaise, cream, and vegetable oils.
Soups	Cream soups made from other foods normally tolerated.
Sweets	Jell-O, gelatin, custard, plain pudding, plain cake, plain cookies, ice cream, sherbet, jelly, sugar, syrup, honey and molasses; and plain candy.
Beverages	Any non-carbonated, non-alcoholic beverage; coffee substitute and decaffeinated coffee or tea.
Spices	Cinnamon, salt, sugar, mace and paprika; flavorings and extracts.

Foods That May Not be Tolerated on Liberal Bland Diets	
Grains	Whole grain cereals, breads, and crackers; pancakes and hot breads; breads and cereals with seeds or nuts
Vegetables	Raw vegetables, potato skins, cooked vegetables that may be gas forming (cabbage, broccoli, Brussels sprouts, cauliflower, onions, garlic, dried peas and beans); corn; peas; and spiced and pickled vegetables, *e.g.,* sauerkraut.
Fruit	Fresh fruit other than bananas or avocados; fruits with coarse skin or seeds; figs; raisins; acidic fruits and juices; spiced or pickled fruits
Dairy	Strong flavored cheese.

Meats and Alternates	Salted and processed meats, and sausages; fried meats, poultry, and seafood. Crunchy peanut butter.
Fats/oils	Spicy dressings.
Soups	Highly seasoned soups; soups with meat based broths.
Sweets	Chewing gum, peppermints, candy with fruit or nuts.
Beverages	Carbonated beverages
Spices/Other	Cloves, caffeine, nutmeg, mace, coffee, chilis and chili powder, tea, cocoa, pepper, and alcohol, coconut, pickles, and olives.

LIBERAL BLAND DIET				
Sample Menu Plan	**Sample Menu**	**Portion Size**	**Nutrient Analysis**	
Breakfast			Energy (kcals)	2305
Grain	White Bread	1slice	PRO (g [%])	96.78 [17]
Grain	Oatmeal	½ cup	CHO (g [%])	271.85 [47]
Fruit	Orange Juice	½ cup	Total Lipid (g [%])	93.72 [36]
Fruit	Banana	1medium	SFA (g [%])	29.769 [11]
Milk	Fat-Free Milk	1cup	MUFA (g [%])	35.906 [14]
Meat	Scrambled Egg Substitute	¼ cup raw	PUFA (g [%])	19.561 [8][
Fat	Margarine	2t	Cholesterol (mg)	258
Beverage	Coffee	As desired[1]	Fiber (g)	18.9
Lunch			Vitamin A (IU)	26956
Meat & Beans	Chopped Stewed Chicken	2 oz	Vitamin E (mg)	12.07
Grain	Soft Dinner Roll	1 roll	Vitamin K (mcg)	147.3
Grain	Steamed Rice	½ cup	Vitamin C (mg)	134
Vegetables	Sweet Potatoes	½ cup	Thiamin (mg)	1.777
Vegetables	Steamed Cabbage	½ cup	Riboflavin (mg)	2.866
Fruit	Canned Fruit Salad	½ cup	Niacin (mg)	26.684
Fat	Gravy	2 oz	Pantothenic Acid (mg)	9.138
Fat	Margarine	2 t	Vitamin B6 (mg)	2.523
Milk	Fat-Free Milk	1cup	Folate (mcg)	272.053
Beverage	Iced Tea	As desired	Vitamin B12 (mcg)	6.1
Dinner			Sodium (mg)	2211
Meat/Beans	Ground beef[2]	3 oz	Potassium (mg)	3899
Grain	White Bread	1slice	Calcium (mg)	1182
Vegetables	String Beans	½ cup	Iron (mg)	19.68
Fruit	Canned Mandarin Oranges	½ cup	Magnesium (mg)	310
Fat	Margarine	2t	Phosphorus (mg)	1494
Fat	Gravy	2oz	Zinc (mg)	13.98
Beverage	Iced Tea	As desired		
Dessert	Cherry Gelatin	½ cup		
Bedtime Snack				
Milk	Custard	½ cup		
Fruit	Canned Pears	½ cup		

[1]One cup was used in the analysis
[2]Some individuals find ground turkey softer to chew than ground beef

HIGH FIBER DIET

INTENDED USE

An increase in dietary fiber is used for the treatment and prevention of constipation. Fiber is also increased for the prevention and treatment of a number of gastrointestinal, cardiovascular, and metabolic diseases. Fiber lowers or stabilizes blood sugar [3,4,5,6,7] and serum cholesterol levels. [8,9,10,11] Some studies have shown that fiber reduces the risk of metabolic syndrome [12,13] and promotes weight maintenance or loss. [14,15]

ADEQUACY

This diet is adequate and meets the Dietary Reference Intakes (DRIs) as established by the Institute of Medicine's Food and Nutrition Board (FNB) for adult males and females.

RECOMMENDATIONS

Fiber may be classified as soluble or insoluble. Soluble fibers are fermented by colonic bacteria and include gums, mucilages, pectin, some hemicellulose, and beta glucan. Soluble fiber is found in fruits, vegetables, barley, legumes, oats and oat bran. Insoluble fibers remain unaffected by digestion and include cellulose, lignin, and some hemicellulose. Insoluble fibers can be found in fruits, vegetables, cereals, whole-wheat products, and wheat bran.

Fiber is found in fruits, vegetables, and whole grain breads and cereal. Meat, dairy, and fats do not contain fiber, so patients should concentrate on having an appropriate intake of fruits, vegetables, and whole grains.

1. The high fiber diet with approximately 20-35 grams of fiber per day is recommended by the Academy of Nutrition and Dietetics. [16]
2. Minimum fluid intake for adults is 2000 mL/day.

Substitution of High for Low Fiber Foods (and Vice Versa)					
Low Fiber Food	Serving Size	Grams of Fiber	High Fiber Substitution	Serving Size	Grams of Fiber
Breads, Cereals, Rice and Pasta:					
White Bread	1 slice	0.6	Whole Wheat Bread	1 slice	1.9
Cooked White Rice	1 cup	0.6	Cooked Brown Rice	1 cup	3.5
Cooked Spaghetti	1 cup	2.3	Cooked Whole Wheat Spaghetti	1 cup	6.3
Cooked Cereal:					
Cream of Wheat Cereal	1 cup	1.2	Oatmeal	1 cup	4.0
Grits	1 cup	0.7	Wheatena	1 cup	6.6
Cold Cereal:					
Cornflakes	1 cup	0.7	All Bran Cereals	1 cup	17.6
Special K	1 cup	0.7	Granola type Cereals	1 cup	5.6
Fruit:					

Apricots	1 apricot	0.7	Pears	1 pear	5.1
Watermelon	1 cup	0.6	Frozen Mixed Fruit	1 cup	4.8
Honeydew Melon	1 cup	1.4	Blackberries	1 cup	7.6
Grapes	1 cup	1.4	Oranges	1 cup	4.3
Pineapple	1 cup	2.2	Raspberries	1 cup	8.0
Vegetables:					
Lettuce, green leaf	1 cup	0.7	Raw Cabbage	1 cup	1.8
Cooked Cauliflower	1 cup	2.9	Cooked Broccoli	1 cup	5.1
Cooked Asparagus tips	1 cup	2.9	Frozen Cooked Brussels Sprouts	1 cup	6.4
Raw Spinach	1 cup	0.7	Raw Carrots	1 cup	3.1
Raw Cucumber	1 cup	0.8	Raw Sweet Green Peppers	1 cup	2.5
Cooked Mustard Greens	1 cup	2.8	Cooked Turnip Greens	1 cup	5.6
Cooked Summer Squash	1 cup	2.5	Cooked Winter Squash	1 cup	5.7
Baked Potato	1 potato	2.3	Cooked Sweet Potato	1 potato	3.9
Meats, Dry Beans and Peas:					
Beef	3 oz.	0.0	Baked Beans	1 cup	10.4
Chicken	3 oz.	0.0	Cooked Split Peas	1 cup	16.3
Egg	1	0.0	Chunky Peanut Butter	1 T	1.3
Fish	3 oz.	0.0	Cooked Black-eyed Peas	1 cup	11.2
Dairy Products:					
Yogurt	1 cup	0.0	Yogurt with ½ oz. mixed nuts	1 cup	1.3

WAYS TO INCREASE DAILY FIBER INTAKE

- Increase intake of fruits and vegetables. Instead of consuming high energy snacks, choose dried fruit, fresh fruit, or raw/cooked vegetables.

- Consume a high fiber cereal or oatmeal for breakfast. Choose cereals containing bran, dried fruit, or a fiber supplement.

- When baking, try substituting white flour with whole wheat flour.

- Substitute whole grains for refined grains. For example, instead of white bread or white rice, choose whole grain bread or brown rice.

- Add frozen vegetables to soups and stews.

- Use beans, peas or lentils to make dips or add them to salads.

- Always be sure that the patient has adequate fluid.

HIGH FIBER DIET

Sample Menu Plan	Sample Menu	Portion Size	Nutrient Analysis	
Breakfast			Energy (kcals)	2045
Grain	Whole grain toast	1slice	Protein (g [%])	100.6 [19.7]
Grain	Bran Flakes	¾ cup	Carbohydrates (g [%])	286.04 [56]
Fruit	Banana	1medium	Total Lipid (g [%])	58.96 [26]
Fruit	Orange Juice	½ cup	SFA (g [%])	14.13 [6]
Meat & Beans	Egg Substitute	¼ cup raw	MUFA (g [%])	25.55 [11]
Milk	Fat-free Milk	1cup	PUFA (g [%])	15.17 [6.7]
Oil	Margarine	1t	Cholesterol (mg)	111
Beverage	Jelly	1T	Fiber (g)	37.2
Discretionary	Coffee	As desired[1]	Vitamin A (IU)	30437
kilocalories			Vitamin E (mg)	19.66
Lunch			Vitamin K (mcg)	273.2
Meat & Beans	Baked Chicken/Canola oil	1 roll	Vitamin C (mg)	181.7
Grain	Whole Wheat Roll	½ cup	Thiamin (mg)	3.69
Vegetables	Shredded Lettuce	1pear	Riboflavin (mg)	4.4
Vegetables	Tomato	½ cup	Niacin (mg)	42.9
Vegetables	Baked Sweet Potato	½ cup	Pantothenic Acid (mg)	19.6
Vegetables	String Beans	2½ oz	Vitamin B6 (mg)	4.35
Fruit	Fruit Salad	1cup	Folate (mcg)	823
Milk	Fat-Free ilk	2t	Vitamin B12 (mcg)	12.3
Oil	Margarine	1cup	Sodium (mg)	2028
Beverage	Iced Tea	1cookie	Potassium (mg)	4813
Discretionary	Mustard		Calcium (mg)	1399
kilocalories			Iron (mg)	31.37
Dinner			Magnesium (mg)	513
Grain	Baked Catfish/Canola Oil	2 ½ oz/2t	Phosphorus (mg)	1892
Grain	Brown Rice	½ cup	Zinc (mg)	25.79
Fruit	Dinner Roll	1 small		
Vegetables	White Beans	½ cup		
Vegetables	Mustard Greens	½ cup		
Meat & Beans	Canned Pineapple	½ cup		
Milk	Fat-Free Milk	1 cup		
Oil	Margarine	1t		
Beverage	Iced Tea	As desired[1]		
Bedtime Snack				
Fruit	Fruit Cup	½ cup		

[1] One cup was used for the nutrient analysis.

FIBER/RESIDUE RESTRICTED DIET

INTENDED USE

The diet is intended for acute phases of radiation enteritis, ulcerative colitis, Crohn's disease, inflammatory bowel disease, and diverticulitis. This diet may also be used temporarily pre- and post-operatively and progressed to a regular diet.

ADEQUACY

This diet does not meet the Dietary Reference Intakes (DRIs) for fiber as established by the Institute of Medicine's Food and Nutrition Board (FNB) for adult males and females. The diet does not meet the MyPlate recommendations for beans and it may be difficult to include adequate amounts of fruit and vegetables in the diet. Fiber should be restricted to 10-15g/day. It is difficult to get the recommended number of servings of grain, fruit, and vegetables into a fiber restricted diet. Without adequate intake of grain—especially whole grain, fruit, vegetables, and dairy it is also difficult to consume the recommended levels of potassium. In addition, many patients on a fiber restricted diet have concomitant conditions that severely limits intake of dairy products; regardless of the level of tolerance, milk should be limited to two glasses to reduce the reside in the diet. If patients are lactose intolerant, lactase can be given, fortified soy milk can be consumed, or calcium and vitamin D supplements can be given.

RECOMMENDATIONS

1   Limit milk and milk products (if not tolerated).
2   Limit fruits and vegetables.
3   Use refined breads and cereals (< ½ gram of fiber per serving.)
4   Use very tender meats.
5   Omit nuts, seeds, beans, and legumes.
6   Refer to the list of selected fiber sources.

Foods Appropriate for a Fiber/Restricted Restricted Diet		
Food Group	**Foods Allowed**	**Foods To Avoid**
Grains	White rice, white and refined breads and cereals (grits, Cream of Wheat), pasta.	Whole grain breads, brown rice, any cereal with nuts, coconut, dried fruit, legumes, cornbread, oatmeal, and graham crackers.
Fruit	Strained fruit juices (no prune), ripe banana, canned fruit without skin, canned orange and grapefruit sections without membranes.	Prune juice, raw fruit, dates, figs, prunes, blackberries, blueberries, strawberries, grapes, pears, pineapple, and rhubarb.
Vegetables	Vegetable juices, cooked vegetables including asparagus, beets, carrots, green beans, mustard and turnip greens, tomatoes, spinach, eggplant, yellow and acorn squash, and potatoes (without skin).	Raw vegetables and others not listed in allowed foods. Legumes may not be well tolerated because of the raffinose and stachycose found in them.

Dairy	2 cups per day, if tolerated. Yogurt, ice cream, all types of milk, if tolerated.	Amounts above 2 cups per day or as tolerated.
Meat	Ground and well cooked tender beef, lamb, ham, veal, pork, poultry organ meats, eggs, and cheese.	Tough cuts of meat, skin, and gristle.
Fats	Margarine, vegetable oils, butter, mayonnaise	Fried foods
Soups	Broths, chicken noodle, chicken and rice	All others
Miscellaneous	Salt, sugar, pepper, spices, herbs, cinnamon, paprika, bay leaves. Plain cakes, cookies, and pies made with allowed foods. Plain sherbet, gelatin desserts.	Caffeine and alcohol (especially wine and beer) increase GI secretions and should be limited.

Diverticulosis/Diverticulitis

Nutritional therapy to treat and prevent diverticulosis is a high fiber diet, which will increase the diameter of the colon and decrease the intestinal pressure .[17,18,19,20] An additional intake of 6 to 10 grams of fiber should be gradually added to the recommended 25-38 grams of fiber per day.

Those with diverticulosis have been discouraged for years from consuming **nuts, seeds, hulls, and foods with small seeds**, including poppy seeds, although these are all good sources of fiber. **There is no scientific evidence for this recommendation and the NIDDK does not recommend that these foods be eliminated from the diet.** [21,22,23]

FIBER RESTRICTED DIET

Sample Menu Plan	Sample Menu	Portion Size	Nutrient Analysis	
Breakfast			Energy (kcals)	1922
Grain	White toast	1slice	Protein (g [%])	97.73 [20]
Grain	Corn Flakes	¾ cup	Carbohydrates (g [%])	262.69 [54.7]
Fruit	Apple juice	½ cup	Total Lipid (g [%])	54.88 [25.7]
Fruit	Canned Peaches	½ cup	SFA (g [%])	15.04 [7]
Meat & Beans	Scrambled Egg Substitute	¼ cup raw	MUFA (g [%])	22.74 [10.1]
Milk	Fat-free Milk	1cup	PUFA (g [%])	12.26 [5.7]
Oil	Margarine	2t	Cholesterol (mg)	175
Beverage	Coffee	As desired	Fiber (g)	15.7
Lunch			Vitamin A (IU)	13038
Meat & Beans	Baked Chicken	2½ oz	Vitamin E (mg)	5.94
Grain	Dinner Roll	1roll	Vitamin K (mcg)	285.7
Grain	Steamed Rice	½ cup	Vitamin C (mg)	151.1
Vegetables	Green Beans	½ cup	Thiamin (mg)	2.29
Vegetables	Yellow Squash	½ cup	Riboflavin (mg)	3.05
Fruit	Canned orange segments	½ cup	Niacin (mg)	34.69
Milk	Fat-freeMilk	1cup	Pantothenic Acid (mg)	7.86
Oil	Margarine	2t	Vitamin B6 (mg)	3.07
Oil	Salad dressing	2t	Folate (mcg)	516.05
Beverage	Lemonade	1cup	Vitamin B12 (mcg)	7.84
Discretionary kilocalories	Sugar Cookie	3 small cookies	Sodium (mg)	2521
Dinner			Potassium (mg)	3552
Meat & Beans	Baked Catfish	2oz	Calcium (mg)	1019
Grain	White bread	1slice	Iron (mg)	21.82
Grain	Pasta	½ cup	Magnesium (mg)	285
Vegetables	Cooked Tomatoes	½ cup	Phosphorus (mg)	1342
Vegetables	Raw Spinach Salad	½ cup	Zinc (mg)	10.42
Fruit	Fruit Cocktail	1 cup		
Oil	Margarine	1cup		
Oil	Salad dressing	2t		
Beverage	Iced Tea	2t		
		As desired		
Bedtime snack				
Fruit	Grape Juice	½ cup		
Milk	Pudding	½ cup		

POST-GASTRECTOMY DIET

INTENDED USE

This diet is used to reduce osmotic activity and delay gastric emptying. This diet is intended for patients who have had a total or partIal gastrectomy or vagotomy and experience rapid gastric emptying or dumping syndrome. In dumping syndrome, the contents of the stomach are transported or "dumped" into the small intestine too quickly.

ADEQUACY

Although this diet *may* meet all of the Dietary Reference Intakes (DRIs) as established by the Institute of Medicine's Food and Nutrition Board (FNB) for adult males and females, patients may have a transient or permanent lactose intolerance and be unable to absorb iron, folate, or vitamin B12 well. Depending on the surgery, patients may have other malabsorption problems. Anemia or bone disease, including osteoporosis, osteopenia, or osteomalacia may result.[24,25,26,27,28,29,30] Vitamin and mineral supplements should be considered.

RECOMMENDATIONS

1. The post-gastrectomy diet encourages increased protein, moderate use of fat, and omits simple carbohydrates to reduce osmotic activity and delay gastric emptying. The progression of the diet should be individualized for each individual. Dumping can occur from 20 minutes to 1-1/2 hours after a meal. If this occurs, avoid lying down 20-30 minutes after a meal.
2. Residents should drink fluids between meals or 30-60 minutes before or after a meal, not with a meal. Drinks should be moderate in temperature if dumping syndrome exists.
3. Meals should be divided into six small feedings. Food should be eaten slowly and chewed thoroughly.
4. If adequate energy is difficult to achieve due to steatorrhea, adding medium-chain triglycerides to the diet or the use of pancreatic enzymes may be beneficial.
5. Increase complex carbohydrate such as bread, cereal, and potatoes.
6. Immediately following gastric surgery, high fiber foods should be limited and gradually added back to the diet as tolerated.
7. Following a gastrectomy, lactose may be poorly tolerated due to a lactase deficiency. Milk and milk products should be gradually added in small amounts to the individual's diet.
8. The diet should be individualized to meet the person's nutritional needs and tolerances/ intolerances.

Foods Allowed or Discouraged after Gastrectomy		
Food Group	**Foods Allowed**	**Foods To Avoid**
Grain	Refined bread, and unsweetened cereal, pastas, potatoes, rice, crackers, starchy vegetables, beans (as tolerated)	Sugar-frosted or sweetened cereal. Donuts, pastries, and muffins.
Vegetables	Fresh, frozen, canned vegetables, as tolerated	Gas-forming vegetables such as cabbage, broccoli, dried peas and beans, if not well tolerated.
Fruit	Unsweetened fresh, frozen, and canned fruits and juices, as tolerated	Sweetened fruits and juices
Beverage and Dairy	Whole, fat-free, 2% low fat milk, buttermilk, yogurt, and cottage cheese. Start with 1/2 cup and check for tolerance. Milk treated with Lactaid. Decaffeinated coffee, tea, and sugar, and carbonated free beverages.	Sugar-sweetened or containing caffeine beverages. Alcohol, chocolate milk drinks, milk shakes, sweetened fruit drinks, and sweetened carbonated drinks
Meat	Lean and medium-fat meat including beef, pork, veal, poultry without skin, fish, cheese, eggs, and peanut butter	Fried and high fat meat including sausage and luncheon meats.
Fats	All in moderate amounts.	Excess use of fats.
Dessert	Unsweetened gelatin and puddings and other desserts made without simple sugars. Plain cakes, vanilla wafers.	Regular cakes, cookies, ice cream, sherbet, donuts, Danish pastries, candy.
Miscellaneous	Salt, herbs and spices, as tolerated. Soups made with allowed ingredients, nuts, or artificial sweeteners.	Pepper, chili sauce, sugar, honey, jellies, and jam, molasses, nuts, and seeds

POST-GASTRECTOMY DIET[1]

Sample Menu Plan	Sample Menu	Portion Size	Nutrient Analysis	
One hour before breakfast (or one hour after breakfast)			Energy (kcals)	2134
Dairy	Fat-free milk[1] or Soy Milk	1 cup	PRO (g [%])	110.23 [20.7]
Breakfast			CHO (g [%])	306.11 [57.3]
Grain	Whole wheat or white toast[2]	1slice	Total Lipid (g [%])	54.68 [23]
Fruit	Peach Canned in Juice	½ cup	SFA (g [%])	15.46 [6.5]
Meat & Beans	Scrambled Egg Substitute	¼ cup raw	MUFA (g [%])	19.00 [8]
Oil	Margarine	1 t	PUFA (g [%])	12.23 [5]
Mid-Morning Snack			Cholesterol (mg)	150.40
			Fiber (g)	136.97
Grain	White toast	1slice	Vitamin A (IU)	12351.07
Fruit	Banana	1 medium	Vitamin E (mg)	213.09
Meat & Beans	Slice of ham	1 slice	Vitamin K (mcg)	255.4
Lunch			Vitamin C (mg)	157.41
Meat & Beans	Baked chicken	2oz	Thiamin (mg)	3.64
Grain	Steamed rice	½ cup	Riboflavin (mg)	3.922
Vegetables	Green Beans	½ cup	Niacin (mg)	31.45
Fruit	Canned Pineapple	½ cup	Pantothenic Acid (mg)	9.33
Oil	Gravy	4 T		
Oil	Margarine	1 t	Vitamin B6 (mg)	12.39
Mid-Afternoon Snack			Folate (mcg)	523.05
Grain	Crackers	6 saltines	Vitamin B12 (mcg)	35.55
Vegetables	Celery sticks	¼ cup	Sodium (mg)	3382
Dairy	Cottage cheese	¼ cottage cheese	Potassium (mg)	4335
			Calcium (mg)	1374.29
Supper			Iron (mg)	28.37
Meat & Beans	Roast beef	2 oz	Magnesium (mg)	597.29
Grain	Toast	Slice toast	Phosphorus (mg)	1703
Vegetables	Mustard Greens	½ cup	Zinc (mg)	11.27
Vegetables	Zucchini	½ cup		
Vegetables	Mashed potatoes	½ cup		
Fruit	Canned mandarin oranges	½ cup		
Oil		2 T		
One hour after dinner (or one hour before dinner)				
Dairy	Fat-free milk[1] or Soy Milk	1 cup		
Bedtime Snack				
Grain	Graham crackers	3crackers		
Fruit	Watermelon	1 ¼ cup		

[1]The patient that this diet is intended for is a post-surgical cancer or trauma patient.
[1]After gastrectomy patients may experience temporary or permanent lactose intolerance. If patients are unable to tolerate dairy, lactase-treated milk, or soy milk may be given. The nutrient analysis used milk.
[2]White bread was used for the nutrient analysis.
Also during the day, patients should be provided with additional fluids to meet calculated needs.

GLUTEN-FREE DIET

INTENDED USE
The gluten-free diet is used to manage celiac disease, celiac sprue, or gluten-sensitive enteropathy resulting from an adverse reaction to gluten, a storage protein found in wheat, barley, rye, malt and possibly oats. The effect of oats is unclear, but most studies suggest that from ½ to ¾ cups of pure oats are well tolerated by most patients.[31,32,33,34,35]

ADEQUACY
Care must be taken to meet the Dietary Reference Intakes (DRIs) as established by the Institute of Medicine's Food and Nutrition Board (FNB) for fiber for adult males and females. Individuals with celiac disease may be lactose intolerant, and thus fail to meet the calcium or vitamin D requirement, without supplementation. Soy milk or calcium fortified foods may be tried. Gluten free grain products are available; however, many are not fortified. Without these products, meeting the grain recommendations is difficult. Depending on the bowel damage, malabsorption of multiple nutrients may occur, and the patient may need a vitamin and mineral supplement.

RECOMMENDATIONS

1) Patients should initially follow a low fiber, low fat, lactose-free, gluten-free diet. This diet is intended to minimize diarrhea and promote healing of the small intestine. Once symptoms improve, patients may slowly add fat, dairy products, and high-fiber foods back to their diet.

2) Patients should follow a strict, lifelong gluten-free diet to repair and avoid further intestinal damage caused by the body's abnormal autoimmune response. Full compliance is necessary, even if the patient is not showing any symptoms. Non-compliance can lead to further damage of the intestinal mucosa, which can cause severe gastrointestinal distress and nutrient malabsorption. However, following a strict gluten-free diet leads to the healing of the intestines and resolution of all symptoms in most cases.

3) Patients should exercise caution when dining out. Discuss with the manager what foods can be eaten and request that meals be prepared on a surface that has not been contaminated by wheat, rye, barley, or malt. Avoid buffet-style restaurants where risk of cross-contamination of foods is high.

4) Patients should thoroughly review all food and medication labels to determine if gluten-containing ingredients are present. The ingredient list on the food label of all foods should be checked for wheat, barley, rye, or malt as well as processed foods or those containing binders. Patients must contact the food manufacturer by phone or email if there are questionable ingredients such as hydrolyzed vegetable protein, vegetable gum, modified food starch, emulsifiers, natural and artificial flavoring, or artificial coloring to

clarify if they are made from wheat, rye, barley, or malt. Barley flavoring and malt flavoring should be avoided completely.

5) Patients should supplement their diets with vitamins and minerals in the first few weeks of treatment due to associated deficiencies of vitamin D, vitamin K, iron, and vitamin B12. B vitamin supplements may be needed after recovery. This is recommended to make up for the amounts of vitamin B in refined grains. Patients should talk to their doctors about vitamin supplements.

Strict compliance with the gluten-free diet is urged to reduce further complications as a result of malabsorption and exposure to gluten, which will cause an inflammatory response in the body.

Food labels must be reviewed to determine if gluten-containing ingredients are present. The food manufacturer must be contacted for product information if there are questionable ingredients such as, hydrolyzed vegetable protein, modified food starch, emulsifiers, natural and artificial flavorings, artificial colorings, or malt flavoring.

Food Allowed on or not Allowed on a Gluten-Free Diet			
Food Group	Allowed	Foods to question	Food to Avoid
Grains	Special Gluten-Free bread and baked products made from tapioca, arrowroot, corn, potato starch, rice, soy, cornmeal, nut flour, buckwheat, millet, flax, teff, sago, sorghum, amaranth, quinoa, and Montina. Bread and cereal products specifically labeled "Glutenfree" produced without contamination from other gluten containing grains. Gluten-free bread mix. Gluten-free crackers. Gluten-free mixes or ready-to eat gluten-free waffles, muffins, and biscuits Gluten-free pretzels Gluten free granola bars. Pure corn tortillas Plain popcorn, plain rice and corn cakes.

Pasta made from rice, corn, bean, potato, soy, quinoa, or other allowed grains. White and brown rice, wild rice, some Oriental rice and rice noodles.

Grits, cream of rice, cornmeal, hominy, millet. Cereal products specifically labeled "Gluten- | Imported "gluten-free" foods. Flavored potato and tortilla chips. Flavored rice and corn cakes.

Buckwheat pasta Commercial rice mixes.

Rice and corn cereals Buckwheat cereals- Note: Pure oats may be allowed in moderation on a gluten-free diet. At this time all oats processed in the US are contaminated with other gluten containing grains and should not be consumed. | Breads and baked products containing wheat, rye, triticale, barley, oats, wheat germ, wheat bran, wheat starch, oat bran, kamut, orzo, couscous, durum, bulgur, farina, semolina (from wheat), spelt, low-gluten flours. Commercial mixes for biscuits, cornbread, muffins, pancakes, and waffles. French bread, crackers, pretzels, Flour tortillas, Bread crumbs. Imported foods labeled "gluten-free" which may contain ingredients not allowed such as wheat starch. Rice crackers made with brown rice syrup.

Pasta made from wheat, wheat starch, durum, semolina, and ingredients not allowed. Commercial pasta mixes

Cream of wheat, farina, |

	free" produced without contamination from other gluten containing grains. Puffed rice, puffed corn, rice flakes, quinoa flakes, amaranth flakes.		barley, Oatmeal, Malt-o-Meal Cereals containing malt flavoring or malt extract, wheat, rye, oats, barley, bran, wheat germ, bulgur, spelt, or triticale Cereals made from low gluten flours.
Fruits	Fresh, frozen and canned fruits and 100% fruit juices.	Fruit pie fillings, dried fruits, and fruit with sauces.	Dried fruit dusted with wheat or oat flour. Fruit desserts, such as pies, crumbles, or tarts.
Vegetables	Fresh, frozen, and canned vegetables. Potatoes, beans, and legumes.	French-fried potatoes (those in restaurants); and baked beans.	Scalloped potatoes (containing wheat flour). Breaded or creamed vegetables.
Dairy	Milk, cream, whipping cream, buttermilk, lactose-free milk, condensed and evaporated milk, soy milk, plain yogurt, aged cheese, cream cheese, processed cheese, and cottage cheese.	Milk drinks, commercial chocolate milk, nondairy creamers, flavored yogurt, sour cream, cheese sauces, and Roquefort and blue cheese.	Malted milk and sour cream made with wheat starch.
Meat, Fish, Poultry, and alternatives	Fresh meats, fish, shellfish, poultry; eggs; dried beans and peas; soybeans; plain peanut butter; and plain nuts	Deli or processed meat, *e.g.* ham, bacon, luncheon meat, sausage, hot dogs, salami, and other cold cuts; imitation crab egg substitutes, dried eggs; soybean and other meat substitutes; baked beans; dry roasted nuts, and some nut butters.	Canned fish or frozen poultry processed with vegetable broth containing hydrolyzed plant protein (HPP) or vegetable protein (HVP) made from ingredients not allowed. Breaded fish or meats, and imitation meats or fish products with wheat gluten.
Fats	Butter, margarine, lard, vegetable oil, cream, shortening. Homemade salad dressings using only allowed ingredients. Mayonnaise made with cider or wine vinegar.	Commercial mayonnaise and salad dressings *Note: Some people may have a sensitivity to distilled white vinegar which is made from wheat.*	Commercial salad dressings with gluten stabilizers or other ingredients not allowed
Soups	Homemade broth and soups, made with allowed ingredients Gluten-free bouillon cubes, broth, or soups.	Commercially prepared broth, bouillon cubes, or soup. Canned soup and dry soup mixes	Most canned soups and soup mixes Bouillon cubes, and broths with HVP/HPP. Commercially prepared soups made with wheat, rye, oats, or barley products

Desserts and sweets	Sugar, most syrup, honey, jam, jelly, hard candies, plain chocolate, pure cocoa, meringues. Most ice cream Sherbet, sorbet, fruit ices, egg custards, gelatin desserts, rice pudding, made with allowed ingredients Gluten-free cakes, cookies, and pastries	Milk pudding, custard powder, pudding mixes. Icings, powdered sugar, marshmallows, lemon curd	Commercially baked cakes, cookies, muffins, pies, pastries, and baking mixes unless designated gluten-free. Ice cream cones. Chocolate bars with crispy rice, cookie filling, malt, or other ingredient not allowed. Chocolate coated nuts rolled in wheat flour. Licorice or other candies made with gluten containing ingredients.
Beverages	Tea, instant or ground coffee, carbonated soft drinks. Distilled alcoholic beverages such as rum, gin, whiskey, vodka, pure liqueurs. Wines and brandies without preservatives. Some soy and rice beverages	Instant tea, flavored and herbal teas, flavored coffees, coffee substitutes, fruit-flavored drinks, chocolate drinks, hot cocoa mixes. Vodka made from grain	Grain beverages, herbal teas with barley. Beer, ale, malt liquors, and lager; cereal or malted beverages. Some root beers and fruit drinks made with barley or barley malt.
Miscellaneous	Salt, pure black pepper, pure herbs and spices, baking soda, cream of tartar, cornstarch, food coloring, food flavoring extracts, mustard, ketchup, monosodium glutamate made in the US, olives, plain pickles, yeast, pure baking chocolate, coconut, tomato paste, aspartame, sucralose, saccharin. Vinegars (apple cider, balsamic, wine, and rice vinegar preferred). Gluten-free soy sauce, Sauces and gravies made with allowed ingredients	Mixed spices and seasonings such as curry powder and chili powder. Baking powder Worcestershire sauce. Bottled meat sauce. Soy sauce. Seafood boil mixes.	Any condiment prepared with wheat, rye, oats, or barley. Soy sauce (made from wheat); imitation pepper packets found in restaurants. Sauces and gravies made with HVP/HPP, wheat flour, oat gum, or other ingredients not allowed. Malt vinegar

Gluten Free Diet				
Sample Menu Plan	**Sample Menu**	**Portions**	**Nutrient Content**	
Breakfast			Energy (kcals)	2237
Grain	Pure Oatmeal[1]	½ cup	PRO (g [%])	95.73 [17]
Fruit	Banana	1 med	CHO (g [%])	328.02 [59]
Fruit	Pear	1 med	Total Lipid (g [%])	65.83 [27]
Dairy	Fat-Free Milk or Soy Milk[2]	1 cup	SFA (g [%])	15.65 [6.3]
Meat	Scrambled Egg Substitute	1 egg	MUFA (g [%])	27.55 [11]
Oil	Trans-Fat Free Margarine	1t	PUFA (g [%])	17.67 [7]
Discretionay Kcals	Jelly	1T	Cholesterol (mg)	148
Beverage	Coffee	1 cup	Fiber (g)	38.5
Lunch			Vitamin A (IU)	39194
Meat/Meat Alternate	Chicken/Canola Oil	2 ½ oz	Vitamin E (mg)	8.28
Grain	Brown Rice	½ cup	Vitamin K (mcg)	698
Grain	Corn Bread (no white flour)	1 sw	Vitamin C (mg)	94.1
Vegetable	Baked Sweet Potato	½ cup	Thiamin (mg)	2.037
Vegetable	Corn	½ cup	Riboflavin (mg)	3.071
Vegetable	Spinach	½ cup/ 2t	Niacin (mg)	23.78
Fruit	Fruit Salad	½ cup	Pantothenic Acid (mg)	9.37
Dairy	Fat-Free Milk or Soy Milk	1 cup	Vitamin B6 (mg)	2.86
Oil	Trans-Fat Free Margarine	1t	Folate (mcg)	559
Beverage	Iced Tea, Unsweetened	1 cup	Vitamin B12 (mcg)	6.4
Dinner			Sodium (mg)	2166
Meat/Oil	Catfish, Baked in Canola Oil	21/2 oz/ 2t	Potassium (mg)	5278
Vegetable	Oven Roasted Potatoes	½ cup	Calcium (mg)	1439
Vegetable	Mustard Greens	½ cup	Iron (mg)	21.23
Vegetable	Black Beans	½ cup	Magnesium (mg)	544
Fruit	Canned Pineapple	½ cup	Phosphorus (mg)	2025
Mik	Fat-Free Milk or Soy Milk	1 cup	Zinc (mg)	11.2
Oil	Trans-Fat Free Margarine	1t		
Beverage	Iced Tea, Unsweetened	1 cup		
Snacks				
Grain	Popcorn	1 ½ cups		
Fruit	Applesauce	½ cup		

[1]Care should be taken to use pure oatmeal and not oatmeals that are processed with the same equiptment as is used for wheat products.

[2]As tolerated.

Additional information on celiac disease and the gluten-free diet can be obtained by contacting the following:

GlutenFree.com
Phone *Inquiries, Orders & Customer Service:* (800) 291-8386

Mailing Addresses
glutenfree.com
P.O. Box 840
Glastonbury, CT 06033

GlutenFree.com also provides an online newsletter with product information and availability, recipes, and other helpful information.

American Dietetic Association Celiac Disease Foundation
13251 Ventura Boulevard, #1
Studio City, CA 91604
Phone: 818–990–2354
Fax: 818–990–2379
Email: cdf@celiac.org
Internet: www.celiac.org
120 South Riverside Plaza, Suite 2000
Chicago, IL 60606–6995
Email: hotline@eatright.org
Internet: www.eatright.org

Gluten Intolerance Group of North America
31214 124th Avenue SE
Auburn, WA 98092–3667
Phone: 253–833–6655
Fax: 253–833–6675
Email: info@gluten.net
Internet: www.gluten.net

National Foundation for Celiac Awareness
224 South Maple Street
Ambler, PA 19002–0544
Phone: 215–325–1306
Email: info@celiaccentral.org
Internet: www.celiaccentral.org

American Celiac Disease Alliance
2504 Duxbury Place
Alexandria, VA 22308
Phone: 703–622–3331
Email: info@americanceliac.org
Internet: www.americanceliac.org

Celiac Sprue Association/USA Inc.
P.O. Box 31700
Omaha, NE 68131–0700
Phone: 1–877–CSA–4CSA (272–4272)
Fax: 402–558–1347
Email: celiacs@csaceliacs.org
Internet: www.csaceliacs.org

Children's Digestive Health and Nutrition Foundation
P.O. Box 6
Flourtown, PA 19031
Phone: 215–233–0808
Fax: 215–233–3918
Email: mstallings@naspghan.org
Internet: www.cdhnf.org
www.celiachealth.org

North American Society for Pediatric Gastroenterology, Hepatology and Nutrition
P.O. Box 6
Flourtown, PA 19031
Phone: 215–233–0808
Fax: 215–233–3918
Email: naspghan@naspghan.org
Internet: www.naspghan.org
www.cdhnf.org

FAT RESTRICTED DIET

INTENDED USE

A fat-controlled diet is used to relieve symptoms of diarrhea, bloating, steatorrhea, and nutrient losses caused when an individual has trouble absorbing fat or that occur when consuming high fat foods.

ADEQUACY

This diet is adequate and meets the Dietary Reference Intakes (DRIs) as established by the Institute of Medicine's Food and Nutrition Board (FNB) for adult males and females. However, if patients are malabsorbing fat, they may not meet the DRI for fat or fat soluble vitamins and may need supplementation with water soluble versions of fat soluble vitamins. Patients may benefit from Medium Chain Triglyceride oil or from pancreatic enzymes depending on their diagnosis. The sample menu here also provides ~ 2000 kcals per day and meets MyPlate recommendations for food groups.

Fat Restricted Diet			
Food Groups	**Servings/Day**	**Allowed Foods**	**Foods to Limit**
Grains	6 ounces; 3 or more of which should be whole grains	Whole grain breads and cereal, enriched breads and cereal, pastas and rice, low fat or fat-free crackers, occasional use of biscuits, pancakes, muffins, French toast and waffles.	Granola or other high fat cereal, high fat chips, and crackers.
Vegetables	2.5 cups	Canned, frozen, and fresh from the following groups as recommended by the DGA and MyPlate: dark green, orange, starchy, dried peas and beans, and other vegetables.	Those cooked in butter, cream sauce, cheese sauce or other high fat sauces. If patient has bloating and diarrhea: gaseous vegetables and dried beans may need to be avoided.
Fruit	2 cups	Canned, frozen, fresh, or dried fruits, and 100% fruit juices (no more than ⅓ of the requirement should be from 100% juice).	Coconut and avocados.
Dairy	3 cups	Fat-free or low-fat milk, buttermilk, evaporated skim and nonfat dried milk, low fat or nonfat yogurt, and ice milk, sherbet.	Whole milk dairy products including whole milk, whole flavored milks, yogurt, cheese, and ice cream.
Meat/Beans	5.5 ounces	Use very-lean and lean meats including loin or round cuts of beef, pork, veal and lamb; poultry without skin; fish, shellfish, tuna canned in water; 95% fat free luncheon meats, egg white and egg substitutes, low fat cheeses; limit whole eggs to 7 per week.	High fat varieties of beef, pork, lamb, luncheon meat, sausage, domestic duck and goose, fish canned in oil, poultry with skin, fried meats, excessive use of peanut butter (which is also high in salt).
Oils	6 teaspoons	Oils, soft, margarine, mayonnaise 1 tsp. = 1 serving Light margarine or mayonnaise, 1 Tbsp. = 1 serving Salad dressing, nuts, seeds 1 Tbsp. = 1 serving, Bacon 1 slice = 1 serving	Fried foods and all fats in excess of 6 teaspoons per day.

Discretionary Calories	With 2,000 kcals, limit to 265 kcals	Jelly beans, gum drops, hard candies, suckers, pretzels, fat-free or low fat fruit bars, graham crackers, ginger snaps, animal crackers, vanilla wafers, angel food cake, Popsicles, gelatin, or cocoa.	All other cakes, cookies, pies, and pastries; puddings made with whole milk or eggs; cream puffs, large amounts of nuts, coconut and chocolate.

2000 KCAL FAT REDUCED DIET

Sample Menu Plan	Sample Menu	Portion Size	Nutrient Analysis	
Breakfast			Energy (kcals)	2160
Grain	Whole Wheat Toast	1 slice	PRO (g [%])	101.06 [19]
Grain	Oatmeal	½ cup	CHO (g [%])	298.42 [55]
Fruit	Banana	1 medium	Total Lipid (g [%])	64.98[27]
Fruit	Orange Juice	½ cup	SFA (g [%])	18.11 [7.5]
Dairy	Fat-free Milk	1 cup	MUFA (g [%])	29.84 [12]
Meat Equivalent	Egg Substitute	¼ cup raw	PUFA (g [%])	20.509 [8.5]
Oil	Margarine	1 t	Cholesterol (mg)	126.00
Discretionary	Jelly	1T	Fiber (g)	30.7
Beverage	Coffee	As desired[1]	Vitamin A (IU)	37021
Lunch			Vitamin E (mg)	12.34
Grains	Whole Wheat Bun	1 bun	Vitamin K (mcg)	662.2
Meat & Beans	Chicken Breast	2 oz	Vitamin C (mg)	124.60
Vegetables	Lettuce, Shredded	½ cup	Thiamin (mg)	2.82
Vegetables	Tomato	2 slices	Riboflavin (mg)	3.079
Other	Yellow Mustard	2t	Niacin (mg)	29.85
Vegetables	Baked Sweet Potato	½ cup	Pantothenic Acid (mg)	9.67
Vegetables	String Beans	½ cup	Vitamin B6 (mg)	2.86
Fruit	Fruit Salad	½ cup	Folate (mcg)	441
Milk	Fat-free milk	1 cup	Vitamin B12 (mcg)	5.29
Oil	Margarine	2t	Sodium (mg)	2250
Beverage	Iced Tea, Unsweetened[1]	As desired	Potassium (mg)	4534
Dinner			Calcium (mg)	1534
Meat & Beans	Roast Beef/Gravy	2oz/4T	Iron (mg)	20.97
Grains	Brown Rice	½ cup	Magnesium (mg)	512
Grains	Dinner Roll	1 roll	Phosphorus (mg)	1741
Vegetables	Steamed Cabbage	½ cup	Zinc (mg)	11.77
Vegetables	Spinach	½ cup		
Fruit	Canned Pineapple	½ cup		
Milk	Fat-Free	1cup		
Oil	Margarine	2t		
Beverage	Iced Tea, Unsweetened[1]	As desired		
Bedtime Snack				
Grain	Graham Crackers	3 crackers		
Fruit	Canned Pears	½ cup		

[1] One cup was used in analysis.

Directory of Digestive Diseases Organizations for Patients

National Institute of Diabetes and Digestive and Kidney Diseases (NIDDK) provides this directory lists voluntary and private organizations involved in digestive diseases-related activities for patients. The organizations offer educational materials and other services.

American Celiac Disease Alliance (ACDA)
2504 Duxbury Place
Alexandria, VA 22308
Phone: 703–622–3331
Email: info@americanceliac.org
Internet: www.americanceliac.org

American Celiac Society—Dietary Support Coalition
Annette & James Bentley
P.O. Box 23455
New Orleans, LA 70183–0455
Phone: 504–737–3293
Email: info@americanceliacsociety.org
Internet: www.americanceliacsociety.org

American College of Gastroenterology (ACG)
P.O. Box 342260
Bethesda, MD 20827–2260
Phone: 301–263–9000
Internet: www.acg.gi.org

Academy of Nutrition and Dietetics (AND)
120 South Riverside Plaza, Suite 2000
Chicago, IL 60606–6995
Internet: www.eatright.org

American Gastroenterological Association (AGA)
National Office
4930 Del Ray Avenue
Bethesda, MD 20814
Phone: 301–654–2055
Fax: 301–654–5920
Email: member@gastro.org
Internet: www.gastro.org

American Liver Foundation (ALF)
75 Maiden Lane, Suite 603
New York, NY 10038–4810
Phone: 1–800–GO–LIVER (465–4837),
1–888–4HEP–USA (443–7872), or 212–668–1000
Fax: 212–483–8179
Email: **info@liverfoundation.org**
Internet: **www.liverfoundation.org**

Association of Gastrointestinal Motility Disorders, Inc. (AGMD)
(formerly American Society of Adults with Pseudo-Obstruction, Inc.)
AGMD International Corporate Headquarters
12 Roberts Drive
Bedford, MA 01730
Phone: 781–275–1300
Fax: 781–275–1304
Email: **digestive.motility@gmail.com**
Internet: **www.agmd-gimotility.org**

Celiac Disease Foundation (CDF)
13251 Ventura Boulevard, #1
Studio City, CA 91604
Phone: 818–990–2354
Fax: 818–990–2379
Email: **cdf@celiac.org**
Internet: **www.celiac.org**

Celiac Sprue Association/USA Inc.
P.O. Box 31700
Omaha, NE 68131–0700
Phone: 1–877–CSA–4CSA
Fax: 402–643–4108
Email: **celiacs@csaceliacs.org**
Internet: **www.csaceliacs.org**

Crohn's & Colitis Foundation of America (CCFA)
386 Park Avenue South, 17th floor
New York, NY 10016
Phone: 1–800–932–2423 or 212–685–3440
Fax: 212–779–4098
Email: **info@ccfa.org**
Internet: **www.ccfa.org**

Cyclic Vomiting Syndrome Association (CVSA)
CVSA USA/Canada
3585 Cedar Hill Road, NW
Canal Winchester, OH 43110
Phone: 614–837–2586
Fax: 614–837–2586
Email: waitesd@cvsaonline.org
Internet: www.cvsaonline.org

Digestive Disease National Coalition
507 Capitol Court NE, Suite 200
Washington, DC 20002
Phone: 202–544–7497
Fax: 202–546–7105
Internet: www.ddnc.org

Gastro-Intestinal Research Foundation
70 East Lake Street, Suite 1015
Chicago, IL 60601–5907
Phone: 312–332–1350
Fax: 312–332–4757
Email: girf@earthlink.net
Internet: www.girf.org

Gluten Intolerance Group of North America (GIG)
31214 124th Ave SE
Auburn, WA 98092
Phone: 253–833–6655
Fax: 253–833–6675
Email: info@gluten.net
Internet: www.gluten.net

International Foundation for Functional Gastrointestinal Disorders (IFFGD) Inc.
P.O. Box 170864
Milwaukee, WI 53217–8076
Phone: 1–888–964–2001 or 414–964–1799
Fax: 414–964–7176
Email: iffgd@iffgd.org
Internet: www.iffgd.org

National Foundation for Celiac Awareness
P.O. Box 544
Ambler, PA 19002
Phone: 215–325–1306
Fax: 215–283–2335
Email: **info@celiaccentral.org**
Internet: **www.celiaccentral.org**

Pediatric/Adolescent Gastroesophageal Reflux Association Inc. (PAGER)
P.O. Box 486
Buckeystown, MD 21717–0486
Phone: 301–601–9541
Fax: 630–982–6418
Email: **gergroup@aol.com**
Internet: **www.reflux.org**

Reach Out for Youth with Ileitis and Colitis Inc.
84 Northgate Circle
Melville, NY 11747
Phone: 631–293–3102
Fax: 631–293–3102
Email: reachoutforyouth@reachoutforyouth.org
Internet: www.reachoutforyouth.org

United Ostomy Associations of America, Inc.
P.O. Box 66
Fairview, TN 37062–0066
Phone: 1–800–826–0826 or 949–660–8624
Fax: 949–660–9262
Email: info@uoaa.org
Internet: www.uoaa.org

RENAL DIETS

INTENDED USE

This diet is intended to provide temporary dietary guidelines until the consulting dietitian can be contacted to calculate the individual's renal diet prescription.

ADEQUACY

This diet does not meet the requirements for phosphorus and, without supplementation, may not meet the requirements for other nutrients contained in phosphorus-containing foods, such as calcium, set forth by the is adequate and meets the Dietary Reference Intakes (DRIs) as established by the Institute of Medicine's Food and Nutrition Board (FNB) for adult males and females. The diet is also low in vitamins C and E, fiber, and magnesium. Diets of patients on hemodialysis are restricted in potassium. Further, since protein restrictions are warranted in some pre-dialysis patients, individuals may not meet the RDA for protein and vitamins and minerals that are contained in foods containing high biological protein, such as iron, zinc, thiamin, and vitamin B12. Patients on renal diets should be supplemented with vitamins and minerals as appropriate.

RECOMMENDATIONS[1]

Condition	Energy (kcal/kg/day)	Protein (g/kg/day)	Sodium (mg/day)	Potassium	Phosphorus	Fluid
CKD Stages 1 & 2	25-35 kcal/kg	0.8-1.4 g/kg	<2400	Usually unrestricted unless serum levels are elevated	Maintain serum values of P and PTH WNL	Not restricted
CKD Stages 3 & 4		0.6-0.8 g/kg			800-1000 mg/day	
Hemodialysis	30-35 kcal/kg (>60 y/o) ≥35 kcal/kg (< 60 y/o)	≥1.2 g/kg SBW ≥50% HBV	≥1 L urine output: 2400-4000 ≤ 1 L urine output: 2000 Anuria: 2000	40 mg/kg IBW or SBW or 2000-3000 mg/day		≥1 L urine output: 2 L fluid intake ≤ 1 L urine output: 1-1.5 L fluid intake Anuria: 1 L fluid intake
Peritoneal Dialysis		≥1.2 – 1.3 g/kg SBW ≥50% HBV	2000-3000	2000-4000 mg/day		Maintain fluid balance

1. If it is difficult for patients to meet the high energy needs, a supplement, such as "Suplena" can be provided.
2. Because fewer kilocalories are being consumed from protein, kilocalories should be obtained from complex carbohydrates and healthy fats such as poly- and monounsaturated fatty acids. If patient has diabetes, eliminate sweets until the diet can be discussed with a dietitian.

3. Foods should be prepared and served without salt or salt substitutes in order to control high blood pressure.
4. In order to reduce phosphorus intake, foods that are high in phosphorus, *e.g.* dairy products, bran cereals, fish and seafood, and dried beans and peas should be avoided. Milk intake should be limited to 4oz daily. Patients can use non-dairy creamer and milk substitutes.
5. In general, fluids do not need to be limited in the early stages of kidney disease. If patients are on potassium wasting diuretics, it may be necessary for the physician to prescribe a potassium supplement.
6. If patient is on hemodialysis and is waiting for a final diet prescription, the hemodialysis diet should be used.

PRE-DIALYSIS--RENAL DIET			
Food Group	**Portion**	**Allowed Foods**	**Foods to Avoid**
Grains 6-8 ounce equivalents[1]	1 slice	Bread (white, French, rye, or sourdough)	Whole wheat bread or crackers. More than 1 serving of cornbread, biscuits, or pancakes per day. Salted crackers, fig bars, gingersnaps, macaroons, cookies made with molasses, oatmeal or raisins, chocolate or nut cakes, Boston cream pie, éclairs, and cream puffs. Whole grain, bran or granola cereals, or wheat germ. Brown or wild rice. Instant commercial pasta or rice mixes.
	½ bun	English muffin, bagel, hamburger or hot dog buns	
	1 6" tortilla	Tortilla	
	½ cup	Pasta	
	½ cup	White rice	
	1 c	Ready-to-eat cereal (Apple Jacks, Fruit Loops, Sugar Pops, Alpha Bits, Cornflakes, Rice Chex, Honey Comb, Sugar Smacks, Corn Chex, Frosted Flakes, Product 19, Rice Krispies, Cheerios)	
	½ cup	Cooked cereal (cream of wheat, cream of rice, grits, Malt-O-Meal)	
	4 crackers	Crackers, unsalted	
	1½ cups	Popcorn, unsalted	
Fruit 1½ cups	½ cup canned, frozen, cut fresh or 1 piece of fresh fruit	All fruit	
Vegetables 2-2½ cups/d	½ cup	Broccoli, cabbage, carrots, cauliflower, celery, corn, cucumber, eggplant, garlic, onion, peppers (all types), radishes, watercress, zucchini and yellow squash. Artichokes, asparagus, avocados, beets and beet greens, collard greens, potatoes, instant potatoes, spinach, winter squash, parsnips, rutabagas, sweet potatoes, yams, low sodium tomato and vegetable juice cocktail, and tomatoes.	Beans, peas, and lentils. Regular tomato or vegetable juice.

	1 cup	Lettuce (all types)	
Milk Limit to one serving/day	½ cup ¼ cup ½ cup 1 oz	Milk (whole, 2%, reduced fat, fat-free) Milk, evaporated Yogurt Cheese	Buttermilk, chocolate milk, commercial milk drink and milk shakes, condensed milk, custard, ice cream, commercial puddings, and cream soups.
Meat	1 oz 1 egg ¼ cup 1 slice ¼ cup	Beef, pork, veal, poultry, and fresh or frozen seafood. Egg Tuna, canned, low sodium Lunchmeat, low sodium Ricotta cheese	Canned salted, pickled spiced, or smoked meats, textured vegetable protein, commercially frozen or breaded fish or meats, nuts and nut butter, and cheese. Dried or canned peas, beans, and lentils.
Oils	1 t	Margarine, mayonnaise, vegetable oil	Salted butter, commercial salad dressings
Discretionary kilocalories	1 t 1 cup 1 T 8 cookies ½ slice	Unsalted butter Carbonated beverages (not diet): Sprite, Seven-Up, Ginger Ale, Root Beer, Kool-Aid, lemonade, Tang, Hi-C, coffee. Sugar, honey, syrup, hard candy, gelatin, popsicles, sherbet with fluid allowance Small sugar cookies Cake, any kind except those with chocolate or nuts.	Molasses, candy with nuts or chocolate. Ice cream
[1]Actual numbers servings depend on the patients' gender, age, and activity level			

0.8 g protein PRE- DIALYSIS RENAL DIET (65 kg IBW patient)
2,000 kcals, 52 gram protein 2 gram sodium 2 gram potassium, 1000 mg phosphorus

Sample Menu Plan	Sample Menu	Portion Size	Nutritional Analysis	
Breakfast			Energy (kcals)	1974
Grain	Cornflakes	1 cup	Protein (g [%])[1,2]	59 [12%]
Grain	White Toast	2 slices	Carbohydrates (g [%])	316 [64%]
Fruit	Grape Juice	½ cup	Total Lipid (g [%])	57[26%]
Fruit	Fruit salad, canned	½ cup	SFA (g [%])	16[7%]
Milk	Milk, whole	½ cup	MUFA (g [%])	23[11%]
Fat	Margarine, unsalted	2 t	PUFA (g [%])	14[6%]
Beverage	Tea	8 oz	Cholesterol (mg)	94
Discretionary	Sugar	2 t	Fiber (g)	14
kilocalories			Vitamin A (IU)	15729
Lunch			Vitamin E (mg)	9
Meat & Beans	Tuna Salad[3]	2 oz	Vitamin K (mcg)	22
Grain	Hard roll (counts as 2)	1 roll	Vitamin C (mg)	62
Grain	Pretzels, unsalted	6 pretzels	Thiamin (mg)	1.698
Vegetable	Carrots, cooked	½ cup	Riboflavin (mg)	20.97
Fruit	Pineapple, canned	½ cup	Niacin (mg)	25.68
Fat	Margarine, unsalted	2 t	Pantothenic Acid (mg)	2.958
Beverage	Ginger ale	8 oz	Vitamin B6 (mg)	2.364
			Folate (mcg)	384
Dinner			Vitamin B12 (mcg)	6.48
Meat & Beans	Hamburger	3 oz	Sodium (mg)	1981
Grain	Hamburger Bun (counts as 2)	1 bun	Potassium (mg)	1896
Fruit	Peaches, canned and drained	½ cup	Calcium (mg)	472
Vegetable	Coleslaw	½ cup	Iron (mg)	19.76
Fat	Ketchup, low sodium	1 T	Magnesium (mg)	175
Beverage	Lemonade	8 oz	Phosphorus (mg)[4]	712
			Zinc (mg)	8.5
Bedtime Snack				
Grain	Apple pie[3]	1 slice		
Fruit				
Fat				

[1]Percent of total energy; [2]58% high biological protein; [3]Many individuals with renal disease also have diabetes; for patients with diabetes, the bedtime snack may be changed to one with less sugar; the phosphorus content of food additives varies among nutrient databases and care should be taken when determining values .

0.6-0.075[1] g protein PRE-DIALYSIS RENAL DIET (65 kg IBW patient)

2,000 kcals, 39 gram protein 2 gram sodium 2 gram potassium, 1000 mg phosphorus

Sample Menu Plan	Sample Menu	Portion Size	Nutritional Analysis	
Breakfast				
Grain	Cornflakes	1 cup	Energy (kcals)	2012
Grain	White Toast	2 slices	Protein (g [%])[2,3]	59.81 [12%]
Fruit	Grape Juice	½ cup	Carbohydrates (g [%])	316.65
Fruit	Fruit salad, canned	½ cup	Total Lipid (g [%])	[63%]
"Milk"	Non-dairy liquid creamer	½ cup	SFA (g [%])	60.82 [27%]
Fat	Margarine, unsalted	1 T	MUFA (g [%])	12.191[5 %]
Beverage	Tea	8 oz	PUFA (g [%])	31.72 [14%]
Discretionary calories	Sugar	2 t	Cholesterol (mg)	13.479 [6%]
			Fiber (g)	285.80
Lunch			Vitamin A (IU)	16.1
Meat & Beans	Egg, hardboiled	1 egg	Vitamin E (mg)	16562
Grain	Hard roll (counts as 2)	1 roll	Vitamin K (mcg)	30.92
Grain	Pretzels, unsalted	6 pretzels	Vitamin C (mg)	38.6
Fruit	Carrots, cooked	½ cup	Thiamin (mg)	81.20
Vegetable	Pineapple, canned	½ cup	Riboflavin (mg)	2.223
Fat	Margarine, unsalted	1T	Niacin (mg)	2.882
Beverage	Ginger ale	8 oz	Pantothenic Acid (mg)	28.094
			Vitamin B6 (mg)	7.089
Afternoon or Bedtime Snack			Folate (mcg)	376
Fruit Supplement	Suplena shake = 4 oz Suplena with 1 T polycose powder and ¼ cup frozen blueberries		Vitamin B12 (mcg)	7.64
			Sodium (mg)	1656
			Potassium (mg)	1999.00
			Calcium (mg)	715
			Iron (mg)	23.21
Dinner			Magnesium (mg)	206
Meat & Beans	Hamburger	2 oz	Phosphorus (mg)	803.00
Grain (x2)	Hamburger Bun (counts as 2)	1 bun	Zinc (mg)	13.85
Vegetable	Coleslaw	½ cup		
Fruit	Peaches, canned and drained	½ cup ½ cup		
Other	Ketchup, low sodium	2 T		
Beverage	Lemonade	8 oz		

[1]Calculations made on 0.75 g/pro/kg. [2]Percent of total energy; [3]37 g of protein from animal sources

RENAL DIET, HEMODIALYSIS

INTENDED USE

This diet is used for the treatment of end-stage renal disease (ESRD) (Stage 5 chronic kidney disease). It is used when kidney function is impaired and the kidneys are unable to excrete the by-products of metabolism which then accumulate in the blood. Sodium, potassium, and phosphorus may also accumulate in the blood, causing the body to retain fluids. This diet helps decrease the workload on the kidneys. Many ESRD patients also have hypertension, cardiovascular disease or diabetes.

ADEQUACY

This diet is not designed to meet either the DRI values for adults or the Dietary Guidelines for Americans. The diets are deficient in calcium, potassium, and phosphorus. Obtaining adequate fiber intake is also difficult since whole wheat products, fruit, and vegetables, including beans, are restricted. Dialysis treatments are associated with a loss of water soluble vitamins; in addition, patients have an increased need for elemental iron. Most patients are on supplements designed for dialysis patients, such as Nephrocaps, which includes the B vitamins: thiamine, riboflavin, niacin/niacinamide, vitamin B6, vitamin B12, folic acid, and pantothenic acid. Vitamin C and calcium supplementation is also needed.

Whole grain and dairy foods should be avoided. Sodium and fluid intake should be individualized and is based on measurement of blood pressure, presence of edema, amount of fluid weight gain, serum sodium level, and dietary intake. There is a small group of dialysis patients that lose, rather than maintain sodium; these patients include those with polycystic disease of the kidney, medullary kidney disease, chronic obstructive uropathy, chronic pyelonephritis, and analgesic nephropathy. In these patients, sodium requirements may be increased to 3 g/day.

RECOMMENDATIONS[1]

Condition	Energy (kcal/kg/day)	Protein (g/kg/day)	Sodium (mg/day)	Potassium	Phosphorus	Fluid
Hemodialysis	30-35 kcal/kg (>60 y/o) ≥35 kcal/kg (< 60 y/o)	≥1.2 g/kg SBW ≥50% HBV	≥1 L urine output: 2400-4000 ≤ 1 L urine output: 2000 Anuria: 2000	40 mg/kg IBW or SBW or 2000-3000 mg/day	800-1000 mg/day	≥1 L urine output: 2 L fluid intake ≤ 1 L urine output: 1-1.5 L fluid intake Anuria: 1 L fluid intake

1. Dietary and nursing service must coordinate the amount of fluid each department provides. Include the fluid contained in nutritional supplements when calculating fluid allowances.
2. Weight variances of 1-3 lbs. before and after dialysis can be expected. Weight gain between treatments should not exceed 4 lbs.
3. Salt substitutes containing potassium must be avoided.
4. Individual and family counseling is important to ensure adherence to the diet. The dietitian will provide the home health agency with a copy of the patient's diet.
5. Meal time adjustments may be required for individuals being dialyzed during meal time. Nursing home residents may bring a sack lunch to be eaten in the waiting room before or after dialysis. Most dialysis centers have an early morning shift and a noon time shift. Some centers have a supper time (evening) shift. It is important to arrange meals so that the patient does not miss needed energy and protein.
6. Phosphate binders such as calcium acetate "Phos-Lo" or calcium carbonate "Tums" are given at mealtime to bind with phosphorus in foods. The phosphorus is eliminated through the stool. Uncontrolled high serum phosphorus levels can lead to serious bone disease. A symptom of elevated serum phosphorus is intense itching.
7. Nutritional supplements such as "Nepro" and "ProMod" powder may be ordered to add energy or protein to the diet.
8. Rice "milk" is low in phosphorus and potassium and may be an acceptable substitute for dairy products by some patients. Non-dairy coffee creamers may also be used.

RENAL DIET--DIALYSIS			
Food Group	Portion Size	Allowed Foods	Foods to Avoid
Grains	1 slice ½ bun 1 6" tortilla ½ cup ½ cup 1 c ½ cup 4 crackers 1½ cups	Bread (white, French, rye, or sourdough) English muffin, bagel, hamburger or hot dog buns Tortilla Pasta White rice Ready-to-eat cereal (Apple Jacks, Fruit Loops, Sugar Pops, Alpha Bits, Cornflakes, Rice Chex, Honey Comb, Sugar Smacks, Corn Chex, Frosted Flakes, Product 19, Rice Krispies, Cheerios) Cooked cereal (cream of wheat, cream of rice, grits, Malt-O-Meal) Crackers, unsalted Popcorn, unsalted	Whole wheat bread or crackers. More than 1 serving of cornbread, biscuits, or pancakes per day. Salted crackers, fig bars, gingersnaps, macaroons, cookies made with molasses, oatmeal or raisins, chocolate or nut cakes, Boston cream pie, éclairs, and cream puffs. Whole grain, bran or granola cereals, or wheat germ. Brown or wild rice. Instant commercial pasta or rice mixes.

Fruit (2-3 servings/d)	1 apple ½ cup ½ cup 10 cherries ½ cup ½ cup 15 grapes ½ cup 1 small 1 half ½ cup 1-2 plums 1 piece 1 small piece	Apple Apple juice/cider Berries Cherries Cranberry juice cocktail Fruit cocktail (drained) Grapes Grape juice Peach (fresh or canned) Pear (fresh or canned) Pineapple (canned, drained) Plums Tangerine Watermelon	Apricot nectar, apricots, avocado, cantaloupe, fresh peaches, honeydew melon, dates, dried fruits, kiwi, maraschino cherries, orange juice, nectarines, oranges, papaya, plantains, prune juice, dried prunes, raisins, and starfruit.
Vegetables (2-3 servings/d)	½ cup 1 cup	Broccoli, Cabbage, Carrots, Cauliflower, Celery, Corn, Cucumber, Eggplant, Garlic, Onion, Peas, Peppers (all types), Radishes, Watercress, Zucchini and Yellow Squash. Lettuce (all types)	Artichokes, asparagus, avocados, baked beans, beets and beet greens, dried or canned beans and peas, collard greens, lentils, frozen lima beans, potatoes, instant potatoes, sauerkraut, spinach, winter squash, parsnips, rutabagas, sweet potatoes, yams, tomato juice, salted and low sodium vegetable juice cocktail, and tomatoes.
Milk Limit to one serving/day	½ cup ¼ cup ½ cup 1 oz	Milk (whole, 2%, reduced fat, fat-free) Milk, evaporated Yogurt Cheese	Buttermilk, chocolate milk, commercial milk drink and milk shakes, condensed milk, custard, ice cream, commercial puddings, and cream soups.
Meat (8-10 ounces/d)	1 oz 1 egg ¼ cup 1 slice ¼ cup	Beef, pork, veal, poultry, and fresh or frozen seafood. Egg Tuna, canned, low sodium Lunchmeat, low sodium Ricotta cheese	Canned salted, pickled spiced, or smoked meats, textured vegetable protein, commercially frozen or breaded fish or meats, nuts and nut butter, and cheese. Dried or canned peas, beans, and lentils.
Fat	1 t	Unsalted butter, margarine, mayonnaise, vegetable oil	Salted butter, commercial salad dressings
Beverages	1 cup	Carbonated beverages (not diet): Sprite, Seven-Up, Ginger Ale, Root Beer, Kool-Aid, lemonade, Tang, Hi-C, coffee	Diet carbonated beverages, Cola-type beverages (Coke, Pepsi, and Dr. Pepper)
Sweets	1 T 8 cookies ½ slice	Sugar, honey, syrup, hard candy, gelatin, popsicles, sherbet with fluid allowance Small sugar cookies Cake, any kind except those with chocolate or nuts.	Molasses, candy with nuts or chocolate.

RENAL DIET--DIALYSIS
2,000 kcals, 80 gram protein 2 gram sodium 2 gram potassium, 1000 mg phosphorus, 1000 ml fluid

Sample Menu Plan	Sample Menu	Portion Size	Nutritional Analysis	
Breakfast				
Grain	Cornflakes	1 cup	Water (ml)	1518[1]
Grain	White Toast	1 slice	Energy (kcals)	2069
Fruit	Grape Juice	½ cup	Protein (g [%])[2]	81 [15.7]
Milk	Milk, whole	½ cup	Carbohydrates (g [%])	292 [56.5]
Meat & Beans	Hard Cooked Egg	2 eggs	Total Lipid (g [%])	66 [28.7]
Fat	Margarine, unsalted	2 t	SFA (g [%])	19 [8.26]
Beverage	Tea	8 oz	MUFA (g [%])	27 [11.7]
Discretionary Kcals	Sugar	2 t	PUFA (g [%])	16 [7]
Lunch			Cholesterol (mg)[3]	538
			Fiber (g)	13
Meat & Beans	Tuna Salad[4]	3 oz	Vitamin A (IU)	15595
Grain	Hard roll (counts as 2)	1 roll	Vitamin E (mg)	10
Grain	Pretzels, unsalted	6 pretzels	Vitamin K (mcg)	22
Fruit	Carrots, cooked	½ cup	Vitamin C (mg)	58
Vegetable	Pineapple, canned	½ cup	Thiamin (mg)	1.67
Fat	Margarine, unsalted	2 t	Riboflavin (mg)	2.60
Beverage	Ginger ale	8 oz	Niacin (mg)	28.28
Dinner			Pantothenic Acid (mg)	4.48
			Vitamin B6 (mg)	2.45
Meat & Beans	Hamburger	4 oz	Folate (mcg)	416
Grain (x2)	Hamburger Bun	1 bun	Vitamin B12 (mcg)	8.93
Vegetable	Coleslaw	½ cup	Sodium (mg)	1798
Fruit	Peaches, canned and drained	½ cup	Potassium (mg)	2018
			Calcium (mg)	483
Beverage	Lemonade	8 oz	Iron (mg)	21
Other	Ketchup, low sodium	1 T	Magnesium (mg)	181
Bedtime Snack			Phosphorus (mg)	961
			Zinc (mg)	11.61
Discretionary Kilocalories	Apple pie[5]	1 slice		

[1]Of the water, 828 ml comes from fluids or foods that are fluids at room temperature--thus, the decisions should be made on how much fluid the patient can actually drink during the day; [2]Percent of total energy; [3]Exceeds cholesterol recommendation--rotate breakfast foods on a daily basis--the menu can be changed to ½ cup egg substitute, this will reduce the cholesterol level to 115 mg, but increases the potassium of the menu to 2306 mg; [4]Made with reduced sodium tuna. Many individuals with renal disease have coronary artery disease, thus cholesterol levels need to be monitored more stringently. The SFA intake for this diet meets the Dietary Guidelines for Americans, but exceeds the Adult Treatment Panel IV recommendations by ~1%. [5]Many individuals with renal disease also have diabetes; for patients with diabetes, the bedtime snack may be changed to one with less sugar.

Additional Information

The National Institute of Diabetes, and Digestive and Kidney Diseases (NIDDK)

HIV/AIDS

INTENDED USE

Good nutrition plays a key role in helping HIV/AIDS patients gain or maintain weight and reduce the complications from infection or medications. [1] Patients can generally tolerate a regular diet (House Diets); however, the virus or antiretroviral therapy (ART) can cause serious medical complications, including metabolic changes such as lipoatrophy or lipohypertrophy, abnormal lipid and glucose metabolism, stroke, loss of renal function, and decreased bone mineral density. [2,3,4,5,6,7,8,9,10,11,12,13] There may be racial and ethnic differences in response to the virus or to ART. [14] Monitoring for these complications and side effects is important since if they occur, patients may need a cardiac diet (Cardiac Management Diet), carbohydrate restricted diet, or renal diet (Renal Diets) or a change in medication to help manage their disease; these diets may not meet the food recommendations of the Pyramid. Patients may also have gastrointestinal complications and may need dietary changes. All patients with HIV/AIDS should observe food safety measures.

ADEQUACY

This diet is adequate and meets the Dietary Reference Intakes (DRIs) as established by the Institute of Medicine's Food and Nutrition Board (FNB) for adult males and females. It is recommended that patients with HIV/AIDS take a multi-vitamin/mineral daily. Additional micronutrient supplementation may be needed; however, this should be determined by the patient's physician. Overall, it remains unclear if supplementation helps patients with HIV/AIDS. If patient with AIDS need to change to specific therapeutic diets, then those diets may not meet the DRI for all nutrients.

RECOMMENDATIONS

1. Energy and protein needs will vary with disease progression and with infection, malnutrition, and renal or liver complications.
2. Three meals per day and between-meal feedings are recommended to ensure adequate intake.
3. Fluid needs are increased with fever, vomiting, diarrhea, and night sweats.
4. Lactose intolerance is common. Often yogurt, cottage cheese, and ice cream are tolerated. Additional protein and commercial supplements are appropriate.
5. Regular monitoring of weight and fat status through bioelectrical impedance analysis (BIA) is important is an indicator of nutritional status.
6. Many antiretroviral medications (HIV medications) cause negative food-drug interactions (Diet and Drug Interaction).
7. Unproven nutrition therapies and megadoses of vitamins are not advised. Multivitamin and mineral supplements providing 100% Daily Value are recommended for all individuals with HIV infection.
8. Many antiretroviral medications contribute to metabolic alterations, including hyperlipidemia and hyperglycemia, as well as body shape changes. Anthropometric measurements should be monitored on patients to determine if changes in diet or medication should be made.

9. Nutrition support may be necessary with a diagnosis of AIDS wasting syndrome.

Nutrition Intervention for Problems in HIV/AIDS Patients	
Problem	**Dietary Modification**
Chewing, swallowing difficulty, mouth/throat soreness or sores, xerostomia	Soften consistency of food to thick liquids or semi-solids. Add sauces and gravies to meals. Use high energy, high protein liquids. Avoid crisp or rough food. Drink liquids with meals. Spicy and salty foods may cause discomfort. Chew sugarless gum or suck on sugar free candies during the day. Rinse mouth with baking soda and water or prescription rinse four times daily. Use artificial saliva.
Nausea or vomiting	Avoid eating in warm rooms. Eat more foods or serve larger meals when the patient is feeling their best. Eat dry toast or crackers upon awakening. Avoid food with strong odors. Provide cold or room temperature food. Avoid food that is spicy or sweet. Eat 6-8 small feedings per day. Avoid favorite foods. Avoid food that is greasy, fried, or high in fat. Provide dry toast or crackers before meals. Sip liquids 30-60 minutes after eating solid food. Sip liquids frequently to prevent dehydration from vomiting. Ask about antiemetics.
Taste/smell changes	Avoid eating in warm rooms. Cold or room temperature foods. Avoid strong flavors or odors. Experiment with seasoning and flavoring to improve tolerance. Strong flavors in tart foods, sauces or marinades may improve flavor. Rinse mouth or brush teeth frequently. If food tastes metallic, use plastic utensils. If patients complain of an intolerance to meats, try adding something sweet, like cranberry sauce or applesauce, or providing other protein sources. To improve smells, drink beverages through a straw.
Anorexia	Provide favorite foods. Adjust meal size to tolerance/adding snacks if necessary. Provide relaxed, pleasant atmosphere. Keep nutrient dense foods on hand, so the patient can respond to hunger immediately. Consider appetite stimulant. Maximize nutrient density. Provide the largest meal when patients appear the hungriest Enteral nutrition or total parenteral nutrition may be warranted with prolonged poor oral intake.
Weight Loss	Provide high energy and protein dense food. Use fortified milk and shakes, whole milk, added sauces, gravies, fat in cooking. Provide commercial or home-made supplements (avoid raw eggs). Encourage snacking between meals. Discourage use of coffee, tea, broth, colas, and other low density foods and

	liquids. Enteral nutrition or total parenteral nutrition may be warranted with prolonged poor oral intake.
Unwanted Weight Gain	Weight gain can be from fluid build-up--a low salt diet may be warranted. Weight gain can also occur from some types of treatment. To minimize unwanted weight gain walking daily as tolerated and if approved by a physician; limit portion sizes of foods eaten; include plant-based foods in the diet; choose lean meats and low-fat dairy products; limit added butter, mayonnaise, and sweets; choose low-fat and low-calorie cooking methods; and limit high-calorie snacks between meals.
Diarrhea	Increase fluid intake to replace loss, but avoid carbonated beverages. Avoid fiber. Low fiber/low residue diet during acute phase. Use soluble fiber such as banana, applesauce, mashed potato, and cooked vegetables. May need to restrict fat or lactose, as needed or treat with pancreatic enzymes if patients report steatorrhea. Eat high potassium foods as tolerated; high sodium foods may also be needed. Avoid foods with sugar alcohols.
Constipation	Increase fluid intake. Increase fiber in diet, as tolerated. Encourage hot beverages. Encourage exercise as tolerated and approved. Limit foods and drink that cause gas. Try to have patient establish a regular stooling pattern. May need stool softener.

FOOD SAFETY

Food poisoning, especially salmonellosis, listeriosis, and campylobacteriosis, can lead to serious complications and death. All food should be well cooked. Proper food handling and safety issues are essential and discussed more fully in the Dietary Recommendations section.

Additional information about HIV/AIDS can be found through the National Institute of Allergy and Infectious Disease (NIAID

CANCER

INTENDED USE

Individuals with cancer usually have increased nutrient needs. Cancer, cancer treatment, and recovery from cancer can increase nutritional needs significantly. Normal digestion, absorption, and metabolism may be affected. Increased protein needs for recovery and repair are usually necessary in cancer patients. A regular diet is appropriate in the absence of gastrointestinal symptoms or other chronic diet-related illnesses. Supplemental nutrition support may be required to maintain or achieve optimal nutritional status and body weight. Modifications might be necessary depending on tolerance, types of cancer, and side effects of cancer therapies.

ADEQUACY

This diet is adequate and meets the Dietary Reference Intakes (DRIs) as established by the Institute of Medicine's Food and Nutrition Board (FNB) for adult males and females. However, additional energy and protein may be needed to prevent weight loss and wasting. Further, some patients with cancer may experience malabsorption depending on the site of the neoplasm or the type of treatment. Radiation to the head and neck area may result in mucositis or xerostomia and radiation to the abdomen can result in radiation enteritis. Chemotherapy or immunotherapy can cause anorexia, taste changes, nausea, vomiting, or diarrhea. A vitamin and mineral supplement providing 100% Daily Value is advisable; however, patients should check with their doctor before taking any medications.

RECOMMENDATIONS

1. Maintaining optimal nutrition is essential for a positive outcome of cancer treatment.
2. Three meals per day and between-meal feedings high in protein are advised to improve intake.
3. Stress a variety of foods to ensure adequate nutritional intake and weight maintenance throughout the continuum of cancer care.
4. Encourage a diet that contains nutrients essential for maintaining health, including protein, carbohydrates (colorful fruits and vegetables), fat, vitamins, minerals, and water.
5. Commercial nutritional supplements are appropriate to increase energy and protein intake.
6. Diet modifications and recommendations need to be individualized for each person's specific nutritional needs and may be necessary to accommodate adjustment to the malignant process and the treatment provided.
7. Individuals with prolonged poor oral intake may be given enteral or parenteral nutrition to prevent wasting.

Information from the National Cancer Association

Surgery may cause fatigue, pain, and loss of appetite.

It is common for patients to experience pain, tiredness, and/or loss of appetite after surgery. For a short time, some patients may not be able to eat their regular diet because of these symptoms. The following eating tips may help:

- Avoid carbonated drinks (such as sodas) and gas-producing foods (such as beans, peas, broccoli, cabbage, Brussels sprouts, green peppers, radishes, and cucumbers).

- If regularity is a problem, increase fiber by small amounts and drink lots of water. Good sources of fiber include whole-grain cereals (such as oatmeal and bran), beans, vegetables, fruit, and whole grain breads. See Gastrointestinal Diets section.

- Choose high-protein and high-energy foods to help wounds heal. Good choices include eggs, cheese, whole milk, ice cream, nuts, peanut butter, meat, poultry, and fish. Increase calories by frying foods and using gravies, mayonnaise, and salad dressings. Supplements high in calories and protein are available. See House Diets section for a high energy, high protein diet.

- Patients with pain may need pain control medications to help improve intake.

Effect of Chemotherapy on Nutrition

Chemotherapy may affect the whole body. Chemotherapy is a cancer treatment that uses drugs to stop the growth of cancer cells, either by killing the cells or by stopping the cells from dividing. Because chemotherapy targets rapidly dividing cells, healthy cells that normally grow and divide rapidly may also be affected by the cancer treatments. These include cells in the mouth and digestive tract.

Nutrition-related side effects may occur during chemotherapy.

Side effects that interfere with eating and digestion may occur during chemotherapy. The following side effects are common: anorexia, nausea/vomiting, diarrhea/constipation, inflammation and sores in the mouth, taste changes, and infections.

Nutrition therapy can treat the nutrition-related side effects of chemotherapy.

The side effects of chemotherapy may make it difficult for a patient to obtain the nutrients needed to regain healthy blood counts between chemotherapy treatments. Nutrition therapy can treat these side effects and help chemotherapy patients get the nutrients they need to tolerate and recover from treatment, prevent weight loss, and maintain general health. Nutrition therapy may include the following:

- Supplements high in calories and protein.

116

- Enteral nutrition.

Effect of Radiation Therapy on Nutrition

Radiation therapy can affect healthy cells in the treatment area. Radiation therapy is a cancer treatment that uses high energy x-rays or other types of radiation to kill cancer cells. There are two types of radiation therapy. External radiation therapy uses a machine outside the body to send radiation toward the cancer. Internal radiation therapy uses a radioactive substance sealed in needles, seeds, wires, or catheters that are placed directly into or near the cancer.

Healthy cells that are near the cancer may be affected by the radiation treatments, and side effects may occur. The side effects depend mostly on the radiation dose and the part of the body that is treated.

Nutrition-related side effects may occur during radiation therapy.

Radiation therapy to any part of the digestive system is likely to cause nutrition-related side effects. The following side effects may occur:

- Radiation therapy to the head and neck may cause anorexia, taste changes[1], dry mouth, inflammation of the mouth and gums, swallowing problems, jaw spasms, cavities, or infection.

- Radiation therapy to the chest may cause infection in the esophagus, swallowing problems, esophageal reflux (a backwards flow of the stomach contents into the esophagus), nausea, or vomiting.

- Radiation therapy to the abdomen or pelvis may cause diarrhea, nausea and vomiting, inflammation of the intestine or rectum, and fistula in the stomach or intestines. Long-term effects can include narrowing of the intestine, chronic inflamed intestines, poor absorption, or blockage in the stomach or intestine.

- Radiation therapy may also cause tiredness, which can lead to a decrease in appetite and a reduced desire to eat. Patients may do well with, multiple small meals or a mechanical soft of even full liquid diet.

Nutrition therapy can treat the nutrition-related side effects of radiation therapy.

Nutrition therapy during radiation treatment can provide the patient with enough protein and energy to tolerate the treatment, prevent weight loss, and maintain general health. Nutrition therapy may include the following:

---

[1] Patients with taste changes may need to be tested for zinc levels which may contribute to taste changes. Other strategies would be preferred foods, and well seasoned foods.

- Nutritional supplement drinks between meals.

- Enteral nutrition.

- Other changes in the diet, such as eating small meals throughout the day and choosing certain kinds of foods.

Patients who receive high-dose radiation or a bone marrow transplant should see a dietitian for nutrition support.

Nutrition-related side effects may occur during immunotherapy.

Immunotherapy is treatment that uses the patient's immune system to fight cancer. Substances made by the body or made in a laboratory are used to boost, direct, or restore the body's natural defenses against cancer. This type of cancer treatment is also called biologic therapy or biotherapy.

The following nutrition-related side effects are common during immunotherapy: fever, nausea/vomiting, diarrhea, anorexia, or tiredness.

Nutrition therapy can treat the nutrition-related side effects of immunotherapy.

If the side effects of immunotherapy are not treated, weight loss and malnutrition may occur. These conditions can cause complications during recovery, such as poor healing or infection. Nutrition therapy can treat side effects from immunotherapy and help patients get the nutrients they need to tolerate treatment, prevent weight loss, and maintain general health.

Bone marrow and stem cell transplant patients have special nutritional needs.

Bone marrow and stem cell transplantation are methods of replacing blood-forming cells destroyed by cancer treatment with high doses of chemotherapy or radiation therapy. Stem cells (immature blood cells) are removed from the bone marrow of the patient or a donor and are frozen for storage. After the chemotherapy and radiation therapy are completed, the stored stem cells are thawed and given back to the patient through an infusion. Over a short time, these reinfused stem cells grow into (and restore) the body's blood cells.

Chemotherapy, radiation therapy, and medications used in the transplant process may cause side effects that prevent a patient from eating and digesting food as usual. These side effects include the following: taste changes, xerostomia, thick saliva, mouth and throat sores, nausea/vomiting, diarrhea/constipation, anorexia, or weight gain.

Transplant patients also have a very high risk of infection. The high doses of chemotherapy and radiation therapy reduce the number of white blood cells, the cells that fight infection. Cancer patients should be especially careful to avoid infections and food-borne illnesses. Patients are advised to avoid eating certain foods that may carry harmful bacteria.

Nutrition therapy can treat the nutrition-related side effects of bone marrow and stem cell transplantation.

Patients undergoing the transplant process need adequate protein and energy to tolerate and recover from the treatment, prevent weight loss, fight infection, and maintain general health. Nutrition therapy is also designed to avoid possible infection from bacteria in food. Nutrition therapy during the transplant process may include the following:

- A diet of only cooked and processed foods, avoiding raw vegetables and fresh fruit.

- Instruction on safe food handling.

- Specific diet guidelines based on the type of transplant and the cancer site.

- Parenteral nutrition during the first few weeks after the transplant is complete, to ensure the patient gets the kilocalories, protein, vitamins, minerals and fluids needed for good health.

Neutropenic Diet

No clear evidence suggests that a neutropenic diet is an independent contributor to reduction of infection in cancer patients or that infection rates are lower in patients on a neutropenic diet as compared with those following standard food safety procedures.[1,2,3,4,5]

Nutrition Intervention for Problems in Cancer Patients	
Problem	**Dietary Modification**
Chewing, swallowing difficulty, mouth/throat soreness or sores, xerostomia	Soften consistency of food to thick liquids or semi-solids Add sauces and gravies to meals Use high energy, high protein liquids Avoid crisp or rough food Drink liquids with meals Spicy and salty foods may cause discomfort Chew sugarless gum or suck on sugar free candies during the day Rinse mouth with baking soda and water or prescription rinse four times daily Use artificial saliva
Nausea or vomiting	Avoid eating in warm rooms Eat more foods or serve larger meals when the patient is feeling their best Eat dry toast or crackers upon awakening Avoid food with strong odors Provide cold or room temperature food Avoid food that is spicy or sweet Eat 6-8 small feedings per day Avoid favorite foods Avoid food that is greasy, fried, or high in fat Provide dry toast or crackers before meals Sip liquids 30-60 minutes after eating solid food Sip liquids frequently to prevent dehydration from vomiting Ask about antiemetics
Taste/smell changes	Avoid eating in warm rooms Cold or room temperature foods Avoid strong flavors or odors Experiment with seasoning and flavoring to improve tolerance Strong flavors in tart foods, sauces or marinades may improve flavor Rinse mouth or brush teeth frequently If food tastes metallic, use plastic utensils If patients complain of an intolerance to meats, try adding something sweet, like cranberry sauce or applesauce, or providing other protein sources. To improve smells, drink beverages through a straw
Anorexia	Provide favorite foods Adjust meal size to tolerance/adding snacks if necessary Provide relaxed, pleasant atmosphere Keep nutrient dense foods on hand, so the patient can respond to hunger immediately Consider appetite stimulant Maximize nutrient density Enteral nutrition or total parenteral nutrition may be warranted with prolonged poor oral intake
Weight Loss	Provide high energy and protein dense food Use fortified milk and shakes, whole milk, added sauces, gravies, fat in cooking Provide commercial or home-made supplements (avoid raw eggs) Encourage snacking between meals Discourage use of coffee, tea, broth, colas, and other low density foods and

	liquids
	Enteral nutrition or total parenteral nutrition may be warranted with prolonged poor oral intake
Unwanted Weight Gain	Weight gain can be from fluid build-up--a low salt diet may be warranted. Weight gain can also occur from some types of treatment. To minimize unwanted weight gain walking daily as tolerated and if approved by a physician; limit portion sizes of foods eaten; include plant-based foods in the diet; choose lean meats and low-fat dairy products; limit added butter, mayonnaise, and sweets; choose low-fat and low-calorie cooking methods; and limit high-calorie snacks between meals.
Diarrhea	Increase fluid intake to replace loss, but avoid carbonated beverages. Avoid fiber. Low fiber residue diet during acute phase. Use soluble fiber such as banana, applesauce, mashed potato, and cooked vegetables. May need to restrict fat or lactose, as needed. Eat high potassium foods as tolerated; high sodium foods may also be needed. Avoid foods with sugar alcohols.
Constipation	Increase fluid intake Increase fiber in diet, as tolerated Encourage hot beverages Encourage exercise as tolerated and approved Limit foods and drink that cause gas Try to have patient establish a regular stooling pattern May need stool softener

Additional information about cancer can be found through the National Cancer Institute and the American Cancer Association.

ENTERAL NUTRITION SUPPORT

INTENDED USE

Enteral nutrition is the provision of nutrients for individuals with a functioning gastrointestinal (GI) tract who are unable to consume adequate oral intake. Indications for enteral nutrition include, however are not limited to coma; dysphagia; surgery of the head and neck or upper GI tract, upper respiratory system, and orthopharynx; ventilation dependence; protein-energy malnutrition; hypermetabolism, including burns and trauma; anorexia nervosa; and central nervous disorders.

Enteral nutrition should not be provided to an individual with severe malabsorption; intractable vomiting; stool output of >1L; intestinal obstruction; peritonitis; paralytic ileus; high output fistulas; GI hemorrhage; or to individuals in the early stages of short bowel syndrome.[2] Before beginning a supplemental feed, evaluate:

1. Premorbid state
2. Current nutritional status
3. Age of the patient
4. Duration of starvation
5. Degree of anticipated insult
6. Likelihood of resuming normal intake soon
7. Unintentional weight loss of >10% in a short period time
8. Serum albumin<3g/100dL

ADEQUACY

Most enteral feeding formulas meet the RDAs and DRIs in 1300 to 2000 ml or when at least 1000 kilocalories are taken in each day depending on the specific formula and nutrient density. A multivitamin and mineral supplement may be necessary to compensate for nutritional deficiency.

RECOMMENDATIONS

1. *Nutrition assessment* by an RD should be completed on all individuals requiring enteral nutrition and should include initial diet history if the patient or a family member is able to provide one; physical assessment; specific nutrient needs; pertinent labs (*e.g.* albumin/prealbumin, complete blood count, electrolytes, glucose, and kidney function); anthropometric measurements; and medical, pharmaceutical, and psychosocial factors that could affect the success of enteral nutrition. See the Nutrition Assessment Section for more specific information.

---

[2] To be fed enterally, patients must have 100 cm jejunal and 150 cm ileal length of functioning small bowel with the ileocecal valve intact for sufficient absorption.

The nutrition assessment should also include the indication of medical necessity for enteral nutrition noting diagnosis that requires enteral feeding and if gravity feeds are not needed, the reason for delivery of the formula via a pump must be included. Acceptable diagnoses for use of a pump include:

- Reflux or aspiration with gravity feedings
- Severe diarrhea unless feeding slowly infused
- Dumping syndrome
- Administration 100ml/hr is necessary for feeding
- Blood glucose fluctuations
- Circulatory overload
- Jejunostomy tube must be used for feeding

A patient must meet 2 basic criteria:

1. PERMANENCE In the judgment of the attending physician and sustained in the medical record, the condition is of long and indefinite duration (ordinarily at least 3 months).

2. FUNCTIONAL CAPACITY The patient's condition could be either anatomic (*e.g.* An obstruction due to head and neck cancer or reconstructive surgery) or due to a motility disorder (*e.g.* severe dysphagia following a stroke).

Additional documentation is required for use of formulas which contain other than semi-synthetic intact protein/protein isolates (elemental or semi-elemental formulas). Disease specific and energy dense formulas must be medically justified. Medicare will not cover enteral nutrition for patients with a functioning gastrointestinal tract whose need for enteral feedings is due to reasons such as anorexia, nausea associated with mood disorder, or end-stage disease with the exception of chronic kidney disease.

B.   Feeding Route

1. Short-term tube feedings (< 30 days) are best with the following placements:
   a. Nasogastric tubes – beginning in the nose and ending in the:
      i. Stomach (nasogastric),
      ii. Duodenum (nasoduodenal), or
      iii. Jejunum(nasojejunal). ...the latter two should be used if the patient is at high risk of aspiration.

2. Long-term tube feedings (> 30 days) are best with the following placements:
   a. Gastrostomy – placed into the stomach through one of the following:
      i. Surgically
      ii. Laparoscopically
      iii. Radiologically
      iv. Percutaneous endoscopy (PEG).

b. Duodenestomy- placed through a percutaneous endoscopy (PEG).
c. Jejunostomy tube – placed into the jejunum through one of the following methods:
   i. Surgically
   ii. Laparoscopically
   iii. Endoscopically
   iv. Needle-catheter jejunostomy (NCJ).

3. Feeding formula should not be administered at chilled temperatures as this may delay gastric emptying and cause GI side effects.

4. Strict hand washing and infection control procedures during preparation and administration of enteral feeding should be maintained. Enteral feeding bags and tubing should be changed every 24 hours.

5. All of the formula in bags should be allowed to finish infusion followed by water flushes before adding new formula. Unless a closed system is used, a formula in a feeding bag should not hang more than 8 hours.

6. Feeding tubes require irrigation every 6 to 8 hours with 40 to 50 ml of water for continuous feeding and after each delivery for bolus or intermittent feedings. Smaller volumes may be used if the patient is fluid restricted. Flushes are also provided when medications are used. Some pumps provide an automatic flush with 25 ml water/60 minutes.

7. Elevate the head of the bed 30 degrees during administration of feeding and at least 1 to 2 hours after feeding has infused.

CLASSIFICATION OF FORMULAS
Formula Selection may be based on many characteristics such as lactose-free, osmolality, nutrient density, kilocalorie: nitrogen ratio, ease of digestibility, metabolic needs, ease of administration, kosher certification, and cost.

A. Polymeric Formula

1. Milk based
   i. Low cost, wide availability
   ii. High residue--may clog small bore feeding tubes
   iii. Adequate vitamins, minerals, and trace elements in limited volume
   iv. Lactose may be difficult to digest by critically ill patients
   v. Bloating, flatulence, cramping, and diarrhea due to lactose may result

2. Standard and nutrient dense
   i. Lactose-free, isotonic, low residue, initiate at full strength (25 ml/hr)
   ii. Inexpensive, easy flow through nasoenteral feeding tubes

iii. Contain intact proteins such as sodium and calcium caseinates or soy protein isolates, oligosaccharides as a carbohydrate source, and long-chain triglycerides (LCT) and medium-chain triglycerides (MCT) as a fat source.

iv. Nutrient dense formulas provide more kilocalories in less volume for fluid restrictions, high calorie/protein needs, or cyclic feedings.

v. 1200 ml usually meets DRIs for vitamins and minerals.

3. Fiber containing formulas
   i. Best for long-term feeding to help prevent gut bacterial translocation
   ii. Blenderized or lactose-free/fiber supplemented
   iii. Fiber supplemented with soy polysaccharides, non-viscous
   iv. May decrease triglycerides, cholesterol, glucose, minimal binding of minerals; may be advantageous in persons with diabetes
   v. May improve diarrhea and constipation
   vi. No decreased mineral absorption with 20-30 gm soy polysaccharides (15-20 gm Total Dietary Fiber)

Benefits of soluble fiber (including pectin, mucilage, gum) and soy polysaccharide:
   a. Increase fecal weight
   b. Increase transit time in colon, delayed gastric emptying
   c. Increase lipase activity
   d. Increase production of Short Chain Fatty Acids (SCFA), a fuel preferred by mucosa which protects against bacterial translocation and protects gut integrity. SCFA's are produced by colonic fermentation of soluble fiber which decreases colonic pH, decreases bacterial proliferation and contributes to sodium and water absorption in the colon.

B. Partially Hydrolyzed
1. Elemental
   i. Minimal residue, low viscosity, minimal digestion required
   ii. Beneficial with malabsorption syndromes, enterocutaneous fistulas, pancreatitis, pancreatic cancer, bowel atrophy
   iii. Crystalline amino acids, oligosaccharides/disaccharides, and vegetable oils
   iv. High osmolality due to formula components

2. Peptide Based
   i. Protein as di- and tripeptides, vegetable oils with MCT oil, and hydrolyzed corn starch or glucose oligosaccharides
   ii. Less hyperosmolar; isotonic

C. Modular Formulas
   Characteristics
       i.   Nutrients such as carbohydrates, protein, and fat are intact or hydrolyzed; powder or liquid
       ii.   May be added to commercial formulas to attain desired nutrient content and manipulation of substrates, especially infant formulas
       iii.   May have physical incompatibilities, especially with nutrient dense formulas
       iv.   No established maximum compatibility to mixing

D. Disease Specific Formulas
   Characteristics
       i.   Specific components to meet needs of disease states such as renal failure, hepatic failure, pulmonary disease, or diabetes
       ii.   Components may include the branch chain amino acids (BCAA), arginine and glutamine which most studies have shown do not improve patient outcome [1-14]

ADMINISTRATION[3]

Each patient's individual case will determine tolerance of feeding, including rate and type of administration. Enteral feeding can be provided as continuous, bolus, gravity, or intermittent feeding.

A. Continuous Feeding
       i.   Continuous feeding involves the gradual delivery of formula by using a volumetric pump
       ii.   It is the preferred method for critically ill patients to initiate enteral feedings and to reduce the risk of aspiration
       iii.   An initiation rate of 25 to 50 ml per hour is advised depending on clinical diagnosis
       iv.   Residuals should be monitored hourly until patient is stable, then every four hours[15, 16]
       v.   If the residuals are less than 150 ml's after 8 hours, advance the feeding rate
       vi.   The feeding may be advanced by 25 ml every 8-12 hours, depending on tolerance and residuals, to meet the goal rate
       vii.   Full strength may be used for most isotonic formulas
       viii.   Diluting formulas may delay the provision of adequate nutrients in a timely manner
       ix.   Hypertonic solutions, such as elemental formulas infused into the small bowel, may be tolerated better at a diluted strength

---

[3] A combination of these methods may be administered in correlation with oral diet or liquid oral supplements. Monitoring the individual's intake via calorie counts is imperative to monitoring for adequate intake.

B. Cyclic Feeding

    i.   Cyclic feedings are also delivered by continuous drip; however time is reduced with an increase in the rate of feeding.

    ii.   This method of delivery is usually delivered during the evening time by pump to facilitate increased intake during the waking hours, for weaning purposes, or to allow freedom to ambulate during the day.

C. Intermittent Infusion

    i.   Intermittent infusion can be infused at specific times during the day when meals are typically consumed (at breakfast, lunch, and dinner).

    ii.   The total volume may be divided into three to six feedings per day.

    iii.   The feeding may be provided by gravity at 200-400 ml over 30 minutes every 2 to 4 hours or over 1 to 2 hours, depending on tolerance and preference to lifestyle.

D. Bolus Feeding

    i.   Bolus feedings may be administered by gravity into the GI tract or by syringe every 4 to 6 hours.

    ii.   The feeding should not exceed 400-500 ml per feeding given over 10-30 minutes several times per day.

    iii.   Feedings of 237- 250 are recommended for best tolerance and to minimize contamination of formula.

    iv.   Bolus feedings may produce and increase risk of nausea, distention/bloating, cramps, and diarrhea, especially in the critically ill.

FLUID NEEDS

- Provide at least 1 ml free water per calorie or 30-40 ml/kg body weight
- Account for other fluids such as IV piggyback, medications, routine IV fluids, and tube flushes
- Account for all losses such as diarrhea, draining wounds, diuretic therapy, and urine output, and replace as needed

---

Quality of Life: It should be noted that adults receiving enteral feeds generally had a poorer quality of life than the control groups. Factors that impacted the quality of life included symptoms such as nausea, vomiting, diarrhea and fatigue. Issues around body image and discomfort while carrying out activities of daily living also impacted the quality of life.[17] Individuals with PEGs had additional issues with leakage and infection of the PEG site.[18] Thus, patients receiving enteral feeds may need additional social support from the staff.

Administration of Medication through Feeding Tubes

1. Medications can be administered through the feeding tube.[19,20,21] Liquid medications, such as elixirs and suspensions are preferred; however if these formulas are hypertonic or contain sorbitol, there is an increased risk of adverse effects, notably diarrhea. Before solid dosage forms are administered, it should be determined if they can be crushed or if a capsule can be opened. Medications should not be added directly to the formula and the tubes should be flushed with 30 ml of water[20] before and after each medication is administered. Bulk-forming agents should not be administered via small bore feeding tubes due to clogging. If the medication is administered incorrectly, it can result in clogged feeding tubes, decreased drug efficacy, increased adverse effects, or drug-formula incompatibilities.

   To minimize drug-nutrient interactions, special considerations should be taken when administering phenytoin.

	Current Recommendation	**Support for the Recommendation?**
Phenytoin	Hold the tube feeding 2 hours before and after administration	Multiple in vitro [22], animal [23], and human case studies [24] have been performed to examine the bioavailability of phenytoin when administered with or mixed with a variety of enteral feeds. A 2000 review was published [25]. Results depended on the form of the drug [26] and the type of the feeding. Randomized controlled trials suggested there was no interaction; however, case studies, although very small, suggested that there was a delay in absorption with break though seizures. Since the consequences of reduced blood levels of phenytoin can be severe, it seems prudent to hold the tube feeds as currently recommended[27] and monitor serum phenytoin levels. This is the ASPEN recommendation[28].

Gastrointestinal Complications		
Complications	**Potential Causes**	**Treatments**
Nausea/Vomiting Note: the feed should be stopped for at least two hours if the patient vomits	Delayed gastric emptying is the most common cause	If delayed gastric emptying is suspected, consider discontinuing or reducing narcotic medications, switching to a low fat formula, using formula at room temperature, reducing the rate to the last tolerated rate or by 20-25 ml and attempt to increase again after 8-12 hours, or administering prokinetic agents, *e.g.* erythromycin combined with metoclopramide. [29-33]
	Improper tube placement	Place tube transpylorically
	Patient Position	Right side to facilitate passage of gastric contents through the pylorus. Head elevated 45 degrees (if possible).
Abdominal Distention	Ileus, obstruction, obstipation, and ascites Rapid formula administration Cold formula	Stop feeding Reduce rate Administer room temperature formula
Diarrhea	Microbial contamination *Clostridium difficile* toxin	Use sterile techniques and infection control measures [34, 35]; decrease hang time to 6 hrs maximum, check *C. difficile* titer and treat with antibiotic therapy if positive. Note that treatment can be refractory and the infection can re-occur. [36]
	Medications Antibiotics Diarrhea –inducing medications, such as magnesium or sorbitol containing elixirs.	Use Ca^+/Al antacids Add fiber to a formula or use a fiber containing formula [37] Administer antidiarrheal medications (loperamide, diphenoxylate, paregoric, octreotide.) Repopulate normal gut flora with lactobacillus granules (one packet via tube, 3 times/day for one day) Change to parenteral nutrition
	Malabsorption	Review patient history Check for malabsorption of specific nutrients; e.g. fat malabsorption may need pancreatic enzymes or lactose maldigestion will need lactose-free formula May need to switch to parenteral nutrition

129

	Hypoalbuminemia Bile salt malabsorption	Increase protein level; switch to parenteral nutrition
	Hyperosmolar formula	Change to isotonic formula
	Lactose maldigestion	Use Lactose-free formula
	Fiber-free formula	Change to fiber containing formula or add fiber to current formula, if tolerable.
	Disease state	Disease specific formulas may help; change to parenteral nutrition with high output stool volume
Constipation	Lack of fiber	Institute a fiber containing formula. [38]
	Dehydration, inadequate fluid intake	Evaluate fluid requirements and fluid provided by formula. Increase water by providing flushes between feedings if intake is not greater than output by 500-1000 mls.
	Drug therapy (pain meds, iron) Reduced gastric motility	Stool softener, alter medications Encourage ambulatory activity Evaluate therapy See above
	Inadequate fiber/bulk	Consider fiber containing formula; evaluate additional fluid needs
	Gastric Obstruction	Stop the feeding, check for impaction

ADITIONAL COMMENTS ON COMPLICATIONS

Diarrhea

Diarrhea has no universal definition, but some have defined it as >500ml every 8 hours or > three stools per day for at least two consecutive days. It is important to evaluate electrolytes (*e.g.* sodium, potassium, magnesium) and to replace as necessary and to monitor I/Os and replace fluid as needed.

Medication, infection of *C. difficile*, contamination, gut integrity, administration technique, malabsorption, and the disease state should be ruled out. The cause of diarrhea should not automatically point to the formula.

Osmotic diarrhea, caused by hyperosmolar formulas, sorbitol, antibiotics, antacids or H_2 blockers, and laxatives or stool softeners may occur. Secretory diarrhea, caused by *C. difficile*; drugs, such as lactulose or intestinal motility, or disorders of the bowel such as gastroenteropancreatic cancer also occurs in patients with enteral feeds.

Types of Diarrhea in Enteral Feeding	
Osmotic Diarrhea	**Secretory Diarrhea**
Hyperosmolar formula	*Clostridium difficile*
Sorbitol	Lactulose
Antibiotics	Intestinal Motility Disorders
Antacids	Partial Bowel Obstruction
Laxatives	GEP Carcinoma--Gastroenteropancreatic
H2 blockers	
Stool Softener	

Metabolic Complications of Enteral Feeding		
Hyperglycemia	Insulin resistance secondary to steroids, stress, sepsis; history of diabetes mellitus or Hyperglycemic hyperosmolar nonketotic coma; dehydration	Insulin administration or oral hypoglycemic agents; use formula with lower carbohydrate content. Use fiber containing formula; change delivery to intermittent feedings to more closely simulate meals. Stop feeding until blood sugar is under control and increase free water.
Hyponatremia	Dilution state-excessive water Excess GI losses- sodium Refeeding Syndrome	Restrict free water; change to a more concentrated formula. Administer diuretics. Replace sodium losses or decrease the rate. Slow rate of feeding
Hypernatremia	Dehydration Free water losses secondary to diabetes insipidus	Appropriate hydration-provide at least 1ml free water/kcal. Monitor intake and output and add free water
Hypokalemia	Diuretic therapy; large dose insulin therapy; increased losses (*e.g.* GI drainage, diarrhea) Refeeding syndrome in malnourished patient	Change to K+ sparing diuretic Give potassium supplementation - Initiate feeding slowly
Hyperkalemia	Metabolic acidosis secondary to renal insufficiency	Use of enteral feeding with low potassium level; correct acidosis with use of bicarbonate solution. Provide kayexalate, insulin, and glucose. Assess renal function

Hypophosphatemia	Large dose of insulin therapy. Refeeding syndrome in malnourished patients. Use of phophate binding antacids	Phosphate supplementation, if phos level is <1.5 Meq, replete by IV. Monitor labs closely. Change antacid. Feed more slowly.
Hyperphosphatemia	Renal insufficiency	Change to renal formula, low in phosphorus; use phosphate binders.
Excess CO2 production Respiratory insufficiency	Overfeeding calories, especially carbohydrates	Provide an enteral formula with balanced carbohydrate, fat, and protein content. Do not overfeed. Monitor phosphorus.
Hypomagnesemia	Refeeding syndrome; alcoholism; malnutrition	Replete with IV magnesium sulfate if <1.0 Meq. Monitor levels.
Hyperalbuminemia	Dehydration	Add free water.
Hypoalbuminemia	Inadequate protein intake	Inadequate protein intake; increase protein; excess urinary or GI loss; volume overload.
BUN	High--Dehydration, kidney failure Low--volume overload, low protein	Add free water, reassess renal function Inadequate protein intake, assess hydration status
Creatinine	High--kidney failure, dehydration Low--low muscle mass	Assess renal function, add free water Depleted muscle mass may be reflected by a low creatinine level.

Mechanical Complications Associated with Enteral Nutrition Therapy		
Complications	**Causes**	**Treatments**
Aspiration-pulmonary	Patient is lying flat	Use appropriate feeding techniques-Elevate head of bed 45 degrees during feeding (if possible) and at least 1 hour following the feeding.
	Poor cough or gag reflexes or unconsciousness	Smaller bore feeding tube; feed transpylorically. Evaluate system of delivery; continuous feeding advised.
	History of Gastric reflux, lower esophageal spincter incompetence or hiatal hernia	Smaller bore feeding tube; change to transpyloric feedings; or administer pro-kinetic drugs.
	Bolus feeding into stomach with delayed gastric emptying.	Monitor gastric residuals. Hold feeding with residuals >100 ml for g-tube and >200ml for NG tube. Recheck in 1-2 hours. A residual of 150-200% of hourly rate for continuous feeding indicates intolerance. Try continuous feedings or prokinetic therapy. Consider concentrated formula at lower rate/volume (although this may cause diarrhea).

	Improper tube placement	Obtain radiological confirmation of tube placement at the time of insertion. Reconfirm placement before feeding by injecting air into the stomach and listening with a stethoscope. Reconfirm placement if patient sneezes, cough violently, or vomits.
Tube obstruction, occlusion, breakage Tube malposition Tube displacement	Causes include small bore tubes, inadequate flushing, viscous formula, but there is no identifiable cause (5% of insertions); excessive gagging or vomiting may also cause problems.	Check tube placement, replace tube, unclog tube. [39-42]
	Acidification	Lubricate the tube by flushing with a small amount of water before and after aspirating gastric residual. Avoid mixing medication with enteral formula. Do not use cranberry juice or carbonated beverages in feeding tubes. [42-43]
	Insufficient tube irrigation	Flush the tube with warm water on a regular basis- before and after each bolus feeding, every 8 hours for continuous feeding, and 30-60 ml before and after medication delivery
	Inappropriate or inadequate crushing of medication through tube	Crush tablets to a fine powder before mixing with water or use liquid form. Use a tube with a large lumen. Use liquid medications as available.

Management of Tube Feeding Complications	
Problem	**Potential Solution**
Clogging the tube	Flush with 20-30 ml of warm water before and after each formula administration; use liquid medications when possible.
Leaking around the tube	Elevate the head of bed 30° upright. Decrease rate if continuous or decrease the amount of bolus feeding.
Vomiting	Stop the feed. Evaluate the cause. After 2-6 hours restart the feed at 25-30 ml less than the last tolerated rate. If vomiting continues, a nasojejunal tube may be necessary or changing to parenteral nutrition.
Diarrhea	Evaluate cause. Consider a fiber containing formula if the patient can tolerate it or consider a formula less hyperosmolar.
Constipation	Evaluate fiber intake and hydration status. Increase free water intake, if the patient is not on a fiber containing formula consider it.
Aspiration	Elevate head of bed 30° during feeding and for 1-2 hours after each feeding has infused; check the placement of the tube--

	for patients at high risk of aspiration, the tube would ideally be placed transpylorically.
Migration of the tube	Reposition tube

It was once recommended that blue dye be added to enteral feeds to help assess the risk of or actual aspiration. The dye should no longer be added to enteral feeds. [43, 44, 45, 46]

Monitoring Selected Laboratory Tests		
	Potential Causes for High Levels	**Potential Causes for Low Levels**
Albumin/Prealbumin	Dehydration--add free water	Inadequate Protein--increase Excess urinary or GI loss--determine cause Trauma or Stress--these are acute phase proteins
Glucose	Glucose intolerance--change to fiber containing formula or lower carbohydrate formula Overfeeding--re-assess energy needs and weight	Hypoglycemia--increase energy, increased complex carbohydrates, fiber, and protein.
BUN	Dehydration, kidney failure--protein in formula may need to be reassessed	Inadequate protein intake--Increase protein. Excess urinary or GI protein loss.
Cr	Kidney failure--protein in formula may need to be reassessed Dehydration	Depleted muscle mass may be reflected by a low creatinine level.
Potassium	Kidney failure Metabolic acidosis can cause a potassium shift	Refeeding syndrome Insulin Vomiting Diuretics
Calcium	Primary hyperparathyroidism Malignancy High Bone turn over Renal failure	Hypoparathyroidism Vitamin D deficiency--including that caused by anticonvulsant therapy, a range of medications, severe acute hyperphosphotemia
Magnesium	Renal insufficiency Decreased intake	Poor dietary intake Refeeding syndrome GI losses--prolonged nasogastric suction, diarrhea, steatorrhea, intestinal fistulas, laxative abuse
Phosphorus	Increased exogenous phosphorus load Decreased urinary excretion Extracellular phosphorus shifts Cellular destruction	Refeeding syndrome Decreased intake Aluminum containing antacids Vomiting Ketoacidosis Diuretics

Also monitor: Weight, I/O, gastric residuals, vomiting, stool output and consistency, intake of formula

Tube Feeding Placement Options

Feeding Option	Comment	Indications	Specific Complications
Nasogastric	Easy access via a soft, flexible feeding tube Tubes are supplied in 8-12 Fr units Anesthesia is not needed	Short term (weeks) Bolus feedings are easier, but continuous feeds are better tolerated	Aspiration[4] Ulceration of nasal cavity Esophageal strictures
Nasoduodenal	Easy access via a soft, flexible feeding tube Tubes are supplied in 8-12 Fr units Anesthesia is not needed	Short term (weeks) Patient at high risk of aspiration	Ulceration of nasal cavity Esophageal strictures
Nasojejunal	Reduces the risk of aspiration	Short term (weeks) where gastric emptying is impaired or proximal leak is suspected Requires a continuous drip	Migration into the stomach Diarrhea is common—in theory a fiber containing formula would help but not well tolerated
Percutaneous Endoscopic Gastrostomy=PEG	Long-term clinical situations Swallowing disorders or impaired small-bowel absorption requiring a continuous drip	Diarrhea is common —a fiber containing formula may help	Requires surgical intervention

Percutaneous Endoscopic Jejunostomy=PEJ	Requires a continuous drip	Long-term clinical situations Gastric emptying impaired or intractable N/V	Clogging or displacement of tube Jejunal fistula if large bore tube used Diarrhea

[1] The risk of aspiration is highest in patients with altered mental status, paralysis, poor gastric emptying, and impairment of swallow and cough mechanisms—particularly patients on respirators

Formula Selection[5]	
No Organic Dysfunction	Standard formula or fiber containing formula; most are moderate protein and moderate energy; and usually well tolerated. They may come in several kilocalorie levels.
Modest Energy, High Protein Needs	Formulas provide moderate energy; but high protein to support lean body mass and wound healing. These formulas are low fiber/low residue.
Diabetes	Reduced fat, modified-fat, fiber containing formula. Some products are consistent with the American Diabetes Association and American Heart Association recommendations and help improve lipid profiles
Renal Formula--pre-dialysis (stage 3 and 4 CKD)	Formulas are available that are low in protein (10% of total energy), high in energy, low in phosphorus and sodium, high in vitamin B6 and folic acid. Some also include 100% of natural vitamin E and scFOS.
Renal Formula--Dialysis (stage 5 CKD)	Formulas are available that meet the altered needs of patients on dialysis and also help to manage blood sugar responses; these formulas are low in phosphorus, potassium, and sodium; high in folate and vitamin B6, and high in protein. These can be used for tube feeding or oral feeding.
Trauma/Stress, Crohn's Disease, and malabsorption conditions	These formulas contain hydrolyzed protein, MCT oil and scFOS. They also can contain EPA and DHA, high levels of vitamins C and E and beta-carotene, and arginine.
For those that are critically ill,	High protein-high energy formulas. These may be supplemented with

[5] For patients on Medicare, disease-specific formulas must be approved.

mechanically ventilated, Those with sepsis, SIRS, ALI, or ARDS	EPA and GLA to modulate information; they may also have vitamins C and E and beta-carotene. Energy is concentrated for fluid restricted patients.
For those that are metabolically stressed with pressure ulcers, multiple fractures, wounds, burns, or surgery	These formulas are energy dense and have high protein. Some also contain a peptide-based semi-elemental protein for easy absorption. Some formulas also include scFOS and arginine.
For patients that are metabolically stressed or immunosuppressed	For those needing a very high protein, energy dense, semi-elemental formula with added immune support agents including arginine, glutamine, omega-3 fatty acids and antioxidants.
For patients at risk for PEM or pressure ulcers	For patients needing high protein and relatively modest energy needs. These formulas may be available with fiber
Ambulatory patients with lung disease or ventilator dependent patients	These formulas are high protein, low carbohydrate, and low fat. Formulas contain high percentage of fat, for example 20%, as MCT oil to enhance fat absorption. These formulas may be fortified with vitamins C and E and beta-carotene.
Patients needing high energy and high protein in a limited volume	These formulas are very protein and very high energy, but have limited fluid. Some products provide
Liver disease	This covers a wide variety problems including hepatic encephalopathy, and the formulas tend to be enriched with Branch Chain Amino Acids (BCAA). The protein needs and the needs for BCCA are very controversial in these patients is very controversial.[44-65]

Note: Both ASPEN and ASPEN have guidelines for enteral nutrition in a geriatric population.[66]

SAMPLE TUBE FEEDING CALCULATION FORM

Patient Name: _____

Tube Feeding Order: (Include Additional Water):

At Goal Rate Feeding Provides: _____ kilocalories, _____ gms protein; _____ ml fluid to meet patient's estimated needs

At goal, does feeding as ordered provide 100% DRIs for all nutrients as appropriate for this patient?   Yes   No

Height: _____ cm   **Weight:** _____ kg

Age (years) ____   **Gender: M   F**

Desirable Body Weight: _____ kg

Mifflin-St Jeor formula

Men: RMR = 10 x weight (kg) + 6.25 x height (cm) - 5 x age (y) + 5

Women: RMR = 10 x weight (kg) + 6.25 x height (cm) - 5 x age (y) - 161.

It's very probable that the activity factor for the population will be 1.2 (sedentary)

Energy Requirements:

Protein Requirements:

Fluid Requirements:

Comments:

Completed By: _____   **Date:** _____

CHILDREN WITH SPECIAL HEALTH CARE NEEDS

Children with developmental disabilities may have special needs that must be addressed in order to provide optimal nutritional support. A child's mental and physical limitations may present problems in all areas of development, including feeding and oral-motor skills. Consequently, a high degree of individualization is needed when assessing the nutritional needs of these children.

Nutrition Assessment

Assessment of the child with developmental disabilities includes all components of nutrition assessment for children without disabilities plus the inclusion of an evaluation of feeding skills and development. A nutrition record is provided at the end of this section to assist with assessment. Taking anthropometric measurements of children who are unable to stand and who have gross motor handicaps may be difficult.

Weight – Weight can be determined using calibrated infant scales, standing balance beam scales, chair scales, or bed scales, depending on the child's involvement. Weight in adults is complemented by body mass index (BMI) measurements; although BMI is the best anthropometric measure of adiposity in children, it is more difficult to assess in children than in adults because of growth and developmental differences. Body mass index-age and BMI percentile may be better indicators in children. A child with a BMI percentile $\geq 85^{th}$ and $< 95^{th}$ is overweight and $\geq 95^{th}$ percentile is obese.[1]

Length or Stature – Recumbent length is measured using an infantometer with a fixed head piece and horizontal backboard, and an adjustable foot piece. The child should be laid in infantometer on top of a pad with the feet toward the foot piece and the head against the fixed. This procedure is best done with two people. The recorder supports the child's head while the examiner positions the feet and ensures that the head lies in the Frankfort horizontal plane. Gentle traction is applied to bring the top of the head in contact with the fixed headpiece. The child's head is secured in the proper alignment by lightly cupping the palms of the hands over the ears. The child's legs are aligned by placing one hand gently but with mild pressure over the knees. With the other hand, the foot piece should be placed so that it rests firmly at the child's heels. The toes must point directly upward with both soles of the feet flexed perpendicular against the acrylic foot piece. To encourage the child to flex the feet, run the tip of your finger down the inside of the foot. When the child is properly positioned, take the measurement.[1]

For other measurements, use recumbent boards, stadiometers, or alternate measurements including arm span, knee-to-ankle, sitting height, or body segments. This is the most useful indicator of growth status and is difficult to obtain accurately. In children less than 2 years of age or those that cannot stand, recumbent length should be recorded to the nearest 0.1 cm according to the recommendations of the CDC. Stature, or standing height, can be measured in children over 2 years of age and should be measured if the child is able to stand. Reliable length of stature measurements may be difficult to obtain in patients with severe contractures, kyphosis or scoliosis. Knee height may be used to assess body length; however, it may not be as accurate in disabled children.[2,3] Upper arm length (UAL) may also be used. In knee height and UAL the

139

right side is usually used unless the child is hemiplegic--then the less affected side is used. The UAL is often used in children with cerebral palsy and reference standards are available for children older than 2 years.

Minimal Time to Detect Changes in Growth[6]	
Measurement	**Interval**
Weight	7 days
Length	4 weeks
Stature	8 weeks
Head circumference	7days, infants 4weeks, up to 4 years
Mid-arm circumference	4 weeks

Head circumference--Head circumference is a useful measurement until approximately 3-4 years of age when head growth slows. It should be measured with a narrow and non-stretchable measuring tape. The child's hair or hair ornaments should be removed to allow for accurate measurements. The measurement is made across the forehead just above the supraorbital ridges, and passes around the head at the same level on both sides of the occiput; the tape is then moved up or down slightly to obtain the maximum circumference. The insertion tape should be perpendicular to the long axis of the face and should be pulled firmly to compress the hair and underlying soft tissues. Record the measurement to the nearest 0.1 cm. The CDC has head circumference charts for boys and girls. If a child has an abnormally shaped head, *e.g.* craniosynostosis, or a low hairline *e.g.* Saethre-Chotzen syndrome, the head should be measured at the largest measurable circumference. Head circumference may be of limited value in children with brain damage.

Skinfolds– Skinfolds can be used to indirectly estimate percent body fat. There are more accurate methods; however, skinfolds are easily obtained, the equipment needed is minimal, and when done correctly correlate well with measurements from hydrostatic weighing. Overall adipose tissue varies among different skinfolds and these are best done over a number of sites. Because it is accessible, the triceps is the most commonly measured skin fold. The measurement is made on the posterior aspect of the right arm, over the triceps muscle, midway between the lateral projection of the acromion process of the scapula and the inferior margin of the olecranon process of the ulna. It is most useful when evaluated over time to assess trends of under- or over-nutrition. To improve accuracy and consistency, children should be measured by the same observed each time. Subscapular skinfolds, can also be obtained, but may be less affected that triceps skinfolds in malnourished patients with neurologic involvement.[4] Triceps skinfolds can be compared with standardized tables.

The World Health Organization has information about and tables to determine percentage skinfold thickness in children. That link also has other information about assessment of anthropometics in children, including training and information on software. The CDC has

---

[6] Adapted from the Pediatric Nutrition Handbook, 6th edition. R. Kleinman, ed. American Academy of Pediatrics. Elk Grove Village, IL. 2009.

140

methodology for anthropometric procedures used in the National Health and Nutrition Examination Survey.

When non-standard methods of assessing anthropometry are employed, careful interpretation is required. Some references such as the Center for Disease Control and Prevention (CDC) Growth Charts, are based on the general population rather than children with special health care needs. There are additional disease-specific growth charts available that might also assist in assessment, *e.g.* Down Syndrome, for premature infants, and quadriplegic cerebral palsy. The CDC also provides information on the growth of children with special health care needs. In spite of the lack of standards for some of these populations, baseline values serve as a control by which changes in an individual's growth pattern may be measured. Additional information on the development of growth charts is available from the CDC.

Clinical and Biochemical Assessment It is important to evaluate both clinical and biochemical parameters. Observing clinical signs of chronic or sub-acute disease and obtaining objective data related to present nutrition status or recent dietary intake will allow for a more complete assessment of the special needs child. Obtaining information related to dental care and disease, past medical history, the child's drug therapy, and laboratory data can help detail the child's nutrition care plan.

Dental Disease Dental caries result from an infectious disease caused by cariogenic bacteria; *Steptococcus mutans* is the most prevalent of these. Dental disease in children may result from structural malformations, oral-motor impairment, tactile defensiveness, delayed weaning, increased consumption of cariogenic foods used by caregivers as rewards, use of cariogenic medications, or poor oral hygiene, as well as drug-related overgrowth or hyperplasia.

From an assessment standpoint, looking into the child's mouth or obtaining information about the mouth can provide both historical and current assessment information; it also helps to identify chewing problems and nutrient deficiencies which help in formulating nutritional goals.

Medical History The majority of these children have significant medical histories. When obtaining the child's medical history, consider prenatal, postnatal, and family history of disease with special attention to areas of nutritional risk. Information surrounding birth history and medical events in the child's life can provide additional information.

Drug Therapy One of the major modes of intervention for children with special needs, including those with chronic diseases, is drug therapy. However, drug therapy is not without complications, and many drugs affect nutritional status.

- Anticonvulsant medications may cause folic acid deficiency (monitor serum and RBC folate), may affect vitamin D status (monitor serum calcium, serum phosphorus, alkaline phosphatase), and may influence the development of hypercholesterolemia (monitor lipid profile).[5,6]

- Drugs for attention deficit disorder may suppress appetite and decrease rate of growth, although this does not seem to be of clinical concern.[7,8]

- Drugs often cause immobility and hypomotility of the gastrointestinal tract and may contribute to constipation which is a major cause of morbidity in children.

Laboratory Data Laboratory values for children with special needs, including developmental disabilities, is generally the same as for children without special needs. Use of medications can alter laboratory values and should be monitored, *e.g.* corticosteroids can elevate blood glucose levels, anticonvulsants can cause dysplipdemia and depletion of vitamin D, and loop diuretics decrease serum potassium levels. Children are subject to many of same problems that adults are, for example re-feeding syndrome, and laboratory values should be monitored in a similar manner.

Dietary Intake When taking a dietary history, it is important to interview all caregivers who are responsible for, or participate in, the child's feeding. It is especially important to differentiate between food offered and actual food consumed, since mechanical feeding problems may result in food spillage and loss. Obtaining a typical day's diet history or a 24 hour dietary recall can be helpful in assessing the child's current intake; however, the problems with 24 hour recalls have long been recognized (underreporting or overreporting may occur). Children often can't remember what they have eaten and parents are not always aware of what their children consume outside of the home. If more in-depth information is needed, the completion of a feeding history questionnaire or obtaining a three- to five-day food record can add supportive data to the child's nutritional assessment. [10-25]

In addition to the above, it is important to evaluate and assess the following:

- Method of feeding (type and special utensils used)
- Persons involved and present during feeding
- Length of time required for feeding
- Level of feeding skills, texture modifications
- Foods causing aspiration or gagging
- Food intolerances or allergies
- Chronic constipation
- Long-term drug use
- Use of food as a reward or pacifier
- Parents' perception and concern about their child's nutritional status.

Behavior and Feeding Skill Development Children with limited means of communication may use their eating behavior to manipulate others in order to gain control over the environment. This type of information can be obtained by observing caregiver-child interaction during feeding and determining whether feeding problems are due to the child's disability, inconsistent management of the feeding situation, food habits, or limitations in the food supply. Common behavior problems include food rejection, tantrums, and other aggressive behavior, such as throwing foods or other objects. Useful techniques for behavior modification include ignoring, time out, continued demand, use of fun and distraction, and shaping.

142

Mechanical feeding difficulties from structural, neuromuscular, or learning abnormalities may include tongue thrust and tonic bite reflex, lack of tongue lateralization, and tactile defensiveness. Once problems are identified, proper positioning, specially adapted feeding equipment, and individual oral-motor therapy are valuable. Types of equipment that may be helpful for food preparation and feeding are:

- Baby food grinder, food processor, blender, vertical cutter mixer for food preparation
- Specialized cups (spouted cup, weighted cup, two handled cup, cut-out cup), specialized utensils (plastic coated spoons, utensils with curved handles) and adapted plates (sloping sides, divided sections, plate guards).

An occupational therapist is a valuable addition to the team assessing children with feeding difficulties.

Estimating Nutritional Requirements In calculating the energy and protein needs for the special needs child, additional needs for activity will be the greatest difference from the normally functioning child. Typically children that are developmentally delayed require less energy per measurement of body weight compared with other children of the same age or size, but will need similar amounts of protein and fluid (more fluid may be required due to inactivity or problems with constipation). When calculating estimated needs for the special needs child there are several methods to use keeping in mind assessment of the child's current nutritional status, *i.e.,* malnourished, stress level, degree of activity. Common methods of estimating nutritional needs are shown below.

Energy and Protein Requirements:

1. Dietary Reference Intakes (DRIs): Use DRIs as a starting point followed by adjustments made using an individualized approach. Adjustments may need to be made based on a child's particular disability. For example, a child with cerebral palsy may need adjustments in the EER (estimated energy requirements) based on muscle tone and altered activity levels. Some children may need less energy while others may need even more energy than the calculated EER for very active PA (physical activity).

Formulas for Calculating Estimated Energy Requirements (EER) (kcal/kg) for Infants and Toddlers[1]	
Age (months)	**Equation**
0-3	(89 x Wt [kg] – 100) + 175
4-6	(89 x Wt [kg] – 100) + 56
7-12	(89 x Wt [kg] – 100) + 22
13-35	(89 x Wt [kg] – 100) + 20
[1]IOM reference	

Formulas for Calculating Estimated Energy Requirements (kcal/day) and Total Energy Expenditure (kcal/day) for Boys[1]	
Age (y)	**Equation**
3 - 8	EER = 88.5 - 61.9 x Age (y) + PA x (26.7 x Wt + 903 x Ht) + 20
9 - 19	EER = 88.5 – 61.9 x Age (y) + PA x (26.7 x Wt + 903 x Ht) + 25
3 – 19, overweight	TEE = -114 – 50.9 x Age (y) + PA (19.5 x Wt + 1161.4 x Ht)

[1]IOM reference
Abbreviations: EER, estimated energy requirement; Ht, height (meters); PA, physical activity coefficient; TEE, total energy expenditure; Wt, weight (kg)

Formulas for Calculating Estimated Energy Requirements (kcal/day) and Total Energy Expenditure (kcal/day) for Girls[1]	
Age (y)	**Equation**
3 – 8	EER = 135.3 – 30.8 x Age (y) + PA x (10.0 x Wt + 934 x Ht) + 20
9 – 19	EER = 135.3 – 30.8 x Age (y) + PA x (10.0 x Wt + 934 x Ht) + 25
3 – 19, overweight	TEE = 389 – 41.2 x Age (y) + PA x (15.0 x Wt + 701 x Ht)

[1]IOM reference
Abbreviations: EER, estimated energy requirement; Ht, height (meters); PA, physical activity coefficient; TEE, total energy expenditure; Wt, weight (kg)

Physical Activity (PA) Coefficients for Boys Ages 3 to 19 years[1]		
Activity Level	**Normal Weight**	**Overweight**
Sedentary	1.0	1.00
Low active	1.13	1.12
Active	1.26	1.24
Very active	1.42	1.45

[1]IOM reference

Physical Activity (PA) Coefficients for Girls Ages 3 to 19 years[1]		
Activity Level	**Normal Weight**	**Overweight**
Sedentary	1.0	1.00
Low active	1.16	1.18
Active	1.31	1.35
Very active	1.56	1.60

[1]IOM reference

Example of Calculating Estimated Energy Intake (EER) and Total Energy Expenditure (TEE)[7]

A WF 4 years, 6 months of age, 105.7 cm tall, and weighs 15.3 kg. She plays outside almost every day, rides a tricycle, and watches not more than 2 hours of television per day. (Use formula for girls 3 to 19 years, active PA coefficient.)

---

[7] Source: CSHCN Nutrition Care Handbook

EER = 135.3 - (30l.8 x age{yr}) + PA x (10.0 x Wt {kg} + 934 x Ht {m}) + 20 = 135.3 – (30.8 x 4.5) + 1.31 x (10.0 x 15.3 + 934 x 1.057) + 20 = 135.3 – 138.6 + 1.31 x (153 + 987.2) + 20 = 135.3 – 138.6 + 1493.7 + 20 = 1510 kcal

Protein Dietary Reference Intakes for Children and Adolescents 0 to 21 Years[1]		
Age/Gender	Grams/day[1]	Grams/kg/day
Infants and Children (both sexes) *Adequate Intake (AI)* 0-6 months	9.1	1.52
Recommended Dietary Allowance (RDA) 7-12 months	13.5	1.5
1-3 years	13	1.10
4-8 years	19	0.95
9-13 years	34	0.95
Girls 13 – 18 years; > 18 years	46; 46	0.85; 0.8
Boys 14 – 18 years; > 18 years	52; 56	0.85; 0.8
[1]AI or RDA for Reference Individual; From IOM		

2. Basal Metabolic Rate x Activity Factor + Disease Co-Efficient
This table is helpful for estimating energy of the special needs child with medical conditions that effect nutrient requirements, *e.g.* malabsorption, respiratory disease.

Calculate Basal Metabolic Rate (BMR) in kilograms using WHO equations		
Age Range (years)	Females	Males
0 - 3	61.0W – 51	60.9W – 54
3 - 10	22.5W + 499	22.7W + 495
10 - 18	12.2W + 746	17.5W + 651
18 - 30	14.7W + 496	15.3W + 679

Calculate Daily Energy Requirement (DEE) by multiplying BMR by activity plus disease coefficients			
Activity Coefficients (AC)		Disease Coefficients (DC)	
Confined to Bed	BMR x 1.3	Normal (lung & GI function)	0
Sedentary	BMR x 1.5	Moderate	0.2
Active	BMR x 1.7	Severe	0.3
		Very severe	0.5
DEE = BMR x (AC + DC)			

Energy Requirements for Specific Developmental Disabilities: Standard methods for determining energy requirements for children with special health care needs are used to begin as an assessment, but alterations may be necessary due to the child's medical diagnosis.

Alternative Methods of Estimating Daily Energy Requirements Based on Health Condition	
Medical Diagnosis	**Energy Calculation**
Down Syndrome	For children ages 5 to 11 yrs: 14.3 kcal/cm for girls and 16.1 kcal/cm for boys
Spina bifida	For children >8 yrs who are minimally active: To maintain weight: 9-11 kcal/cm or 50% fewer kcal than recommended for a child of the same age without the condition and to promote weight loss: 7 kcal/cm
Prader-Willi syndrome	For all children and adolescents: 10-11 kcal/cm to maintain growth within a growth channel And 8.5 kcal/cm for slow weight loss and support linear growth
Children with very low energy needs	• Lower: 7-9 kcal/cm • Moderate: 9-11 kcal/cm • High: 12-15 kcal/cm
Failure to thrive	Will depend on etiology or medical condition, but start with EER calculations using ideal body weight for height-age and EER for height-age.
Cystic fibrosis	Calculate ideal weight based on height, using the pediatric growth chart. Multiply by the child's EER for age. Multiply by a factor of 1.3 – 1.5 (depending on the severity of the disease) to compensate for increased energy demands.

Example: 9 month old girl with weight of 6.4 kg and length of 66 cm (height-age = 6 months). Ideal body weight for a 6 month old girl is 7.3 kg EER (kcal) = (89 x Wt {kg} – 100) + 56
$$= (89 \times 7.3 - 100) + 56 = 550 + 56 = 606 \text{ kcals}[8]$$

In addition, requirements of children and adolescents with cerebral palsy appear to be disease-specific and varying depending on functional capacity, degree of mobility, severity of disease, and level of altered metabolism .[26] For example, children with spastic quadriplegic cerebral palsy usually require 1.1 x measured REE.[27]

Catch-up Growth Requirements: The following calculations may overestimate needs in non-ambulatory children with a decreased level of activity due to motor dysfunction. Caution must be exercised when attempting to apply "rule-of-thumb principles" in this population. A high degree of individualization and tailoring of nutrition care plans based on monitored response to nutrition therapy is needed for children with developmental disabilities.

Estimating energy and protein needs for catch-up growth:[9]

Kcal/kg = <u>Ideal weight for height x RDA kcal/kg Height age</u>
                           Actual weight

---

[8] Source: CSHCN Nutrition Care Handbook

[9] Source: Karen Yowell-Warman and Patricia Queen. "Pediatric Nutrition in the Home." In Mindy Hermann-Zandins and Riva Touger Decker, eds. *Nutrition Support in Home Health*. Aspen Publishers, Inc., © 1989.

Growth Velocity

Weight increase Age (g/day)

0-3 months 25-35 g/d
3-6 months 15-21 g/g
6-12 months 10-13 g/d
1-6 years 5-8   g/d
7-10 years 5-11   g/d

Growth suppression can occur as a result of under nutrition or illness. During the recovery phase, a child can grow at a rate greater than that expected for age.
As the more rapid growth proceeds, the child "catches up" to his or her growth curve.
Source: *American Journal of Clinical Nutrition*. Vol 35 pp. 1169-1175. American Society for Clinical Nutrition, Inc. © 1982.

$$\text{Protein (g/kg)} = \frac{\text{Ideal weight for height x RDA protein (g/kg) Height Age}}{\text{Actual weight}}$$

Reference Standards for Growth

Once nutrition intervention has been initiated the following standards will help in the assessment of the child's growth and provide information in regard to nutritional goals for the child. Once catch-up growth has been achieved weight gain goals per day should decrease so the child will not become obese. Periodic assessment of the child's growth is imperative in order to achieve a good nutritional status.

Fluid Requirements Providing the necessary fluids to the child with special needs is essential to their nutritional care. Needs will vary but all children will, at least, require the appropriate amount of fluids to meet maintenance needs. Excessive sweating and constipation for example will increase the fluid requirements for a child.

Recommended Fluid Intake	
Child's Weight	**Total Fluids Needed in 24 hours**
7 lb	2 cups
12 lb	3 1/3 cups
21 lb	5 cups
26 lb	6 cups
36 lb	7 cups
44 lb	8 cups
By body weight: 1,500 – 1,800 ml/m2/day	
Body Maintenance Fluid Needs Per Day Weight	
1-10 kg 100 ml/kg 11-20 kg 1,000 ml plus 50 ml for each kg > 10 kg >20 kg 1,500 ml plus 20 ml for each kg > 20 kg Average fluid intake is 1 ½ to 2 times maintenance needs. Source: Reprinted from *Manual of Pediatric Parenteral Nutrition* by J. A. Kerner, with permission of Churchill-Livingstone, Inc. ©1983	

The total water requirements for infants, children, and adolescents from the Institute of Medicine are:

Infants
0-6 mo 0.7 L/day
712 mo 0.8 L/day

Males
9-13 y 2.4 L/day
14-18 y 3.3 L/day

Children
1-3 y 1.3 L/day
4-8 y 1.7 L/day

Females
9-13 y 2.1 L/day
14-18 y 2.3 L/day

Common Nutritional Problems for the Special Needs Child			
Problems:	**May Result From:**	**May result In:**	**Treatment Goal:**
Feeding problems	Handicapping conditions Down Syndrome Cleft palate Cerebral Palsy Loss of Limbs Epilepsy Dysphagia	Malnutrition	Proper positioning Proper utensils Assistance by staff Modified food texture
Marked weight gain	Inactivity Increased consumption of high energy foods Some medication Down Syndrome Spina Bifida Prader-Willi Syndrome	Obesity Poor motor development Poor self-image	Decreased rate of weight gain
Marked weight loss	Growth slowdown Severe illness/diarrhea/vomiting Malabsorption Refusal to eat Congenital heart disease Atheoid cerebral palsy	Severe malnutrition	Identify cause Increase weight slowly
Refusal to eat or prolonged anorexia	Foods of incorrect texture Severe illness Behavioral problems Poor positioning Tiredness Sensitive mouth area Medications	Marked weight loss Malnutrition	Identify cause Increase weight slowly Overcome causes of poor eating Refer to OT Refer to psychologist
Gagging/vomiting/rumination	Sensitive mouth area Attention-getting behavior Food passage blocked	Malnutrition	Change texture of food Refer to speech Refer to OT Ignore or use

			behavior modification
Constipation	Down Syndrome Spastic cerebral palsy Inactivity Lack of fiber in diet Medications	Severe abdominal pain and bleeding Anorexia	Increase activity Increase fluid Increase fiber
Diarrhea or vomiting	Improper feeding Viral infection Digestive problem Stress Food poisoning Medications Allergy	Dehydration Weight loss	Identify cause Diet change Encourage fluids
Excessive fluid loss or intake of fluids	Dysphagia Medications Vomiting or diarrhea	Dehydration	Refer to Speech Encourage fluids Physician examination
Medication/Food Interaction	Anticonvulsants Tranquilizers Stimulants Antibiotics Antidepressants/antimanics ADHD	Vitamin/mineral deficiencies Dental/gum problems Constipation Anorexia Weight loss	Diet appropriate to the medication Increase fiber and fluid Increase weight slowly
Pica	Increased need to suck Emotional factors Mental retardation	Lead poisoning Anemia Learning problems	Psychologist consult Assess nutritional needs
Dental problems	Poor oral hygiene Frequent sugary snacks Poor tooth enamel Tranquilizer use	Poor chewing Pain	Good oral hygiene Decrease cariogenic foods
Adapted From: Lois Schmidt. "Nutrition for Children with Special Needs." Adapted from School Nutrition and Food Service Techniques for Children with Exceptional Needs. California State Department of Education. Office of Child Nutrition, United Cerebral Palsy of Minnesota, 1985.			

Supplemental Nutrition Support[28,29,30]

Enteral nutrition is preferred over parenteral nutrition since it reduces the number of metabolic and infectious complications, provides prophylaxis against stress-induced gastropathy and gastrointestinal hemorrhage, and provides a trophic effect on the gut.

Conditions in which enteral feeds may be warranted[10]	
Cardiorespiratory illness	Protracted or high volume diarrhea
Chronic lung disease	Renal disease
Cystic fibrosis	Hypermetabolic states--including burn injury, severe trauma, or closed head injury
Congenital heart disease	Cancer
Gastrointestinal tract disease	Neurological disease
Inflammatory bowel disease	Cerebral palsy
Short bowel syndrome	Oral motor dysfunction
Biliary atresia	Prolonged inadequate intake
Gastrointestinal reflux	Dysphagia
Renal disease	Malnutrition

If children or adolescents can swallow, prior to tube feeding, try offering them the formulas p.o. All purpose pediatric formulas usually come in oral supplement and tube feeding "versions" or the enteral formula can be used as a p.o. supplement.

Two vendors sell pediatric enteral formulas for children 1 to 10 years of age. The energy distribution of protein, carbohydrates, and fats are between those required by infants and by adults. Most formulas meet or exceed the RDA for micronutrients if provided in volumes of 950 to 1200 ml. Children 10 years of age and older or those with needing disease-specific formulas can generally have an adult formula. It's possible that some disease-specific formulas, especially the ones with high energy density may exceed the renal solute capability and may lead to diarrhea, vomiting, abdominal distention, and delayed gastric emptying. These formulas may need to be diluted for young children; however, this will also dilute the nutrients, so care should be taken.

Formula selection depends on the caloric density, nutrient composition and source, digestibility, accessibility, viscosity, osmolality, and cost. In most situations, the use of fiber-containing formulas is recommended since the majority of these children have poor intestinal motility resulting in constipation. Elemental or semi-elemental formulas do not provide an advantage if the child has normal digestive function. Evaluation of formula selection should be ongoing to determine its appropriateness to the changing needs of the infant, child, or adolescent.

---

[10] Adapted from Walker AW, Kleinman RE, Sherman PM, Sanderson IR, Goulet O, Shneider BL (eds). Pediatric Gastrointestinal Disease. 2nd edition. Burlington, Ontario: BC Decker, Inc. 1995

ADVERSE REACTIONS TO FOOD

Adverse reactions to food include food intolerances and food allerigies. Food intolerances can include responses to pharmacologic agents or bacterial toxins, and non-toxic reactions resulting from enzyme deficiencies, inborn errors of metabolism, or non-reproducible adverse reactions. Food allergies are also known as Immunoglobulin E (IgE) immune reactions. Other diseases that can be confused with a food allergy include celiac disease, gustatory rhinitis, irritable bowel syndrome, and anorexia nervosa.[1]

The Joint Commission requires that information about food allergies be placed in an in-patient's chart. For in-patients in long term care facilities, The Joint Commission standards and elements of performance require that dietary and food allergies are assessed . In acute care and long term care facilities it is critical that the food service staff and nursing staff be alerted to any patients with food allergies in order to avoid cross contaminating food or utensils or serving the patient these foods. In addition, for patients with food allergies or idiopathic anaphylaxis, a consult with a licensed dietitian/nutritionist should assess dietary intake and assure that the patient is appropriately counseled to avoid food-allergic reactions after discharge. Idiopathic anaphylaxis can result from food allergens to masked or hidden foods.

Food allergies occur within minutes up to two hours after exposure to the food. Allergic reactions commonly express themselves through gastrointestinal (*e.g.* cramping, vomiting, and diarrhea), respiratory (*e.g.* asthma, rhinitis), and cutaneous symptoms (*e.g.* eczema, pruritis, urticaria) and oral allergy syndrome (*e.g.* pruritus and burning of the oral cavity; angioedema of the lips, tongue, or oropharynx). Anaphylaxis is a multisystemic reaction, characterized by hypotension, shock, cramping, diarrhea, vomiting, generalized urticaria, dyspnea, wheezing, swelling of the throat, and a feeling of impending doom. This is a medical emergency. [1]

Most food allergies develop in childhood, although they can develop at any age. In theory any food can elicit a food allergy; however, in infants and children, the most common food allergies are to cow's milk, egg, peanut, wheat, soy, tree nuts, finned fish, and shellfish.[1] Allergies to milk, egg, soy, and wheat usually resolve; peanut, tree nut, and seafood allergies generally do not.[2] Currently, the only ways to manage food allergies is to avoid the allergen and initiate therapy for an allergic reaction if ingestion does occur. Severe allergic reactions are medical emergencies.

For in- or out-patients with food allergies, nutrient and fluid requirements are the same as for individuals without food allergies. Since individuals with adverse reactions to food may self-restrict intake or have been counseled on food avoidance, it is particularly important to determine dietary adequacy and to provide individuals with appropriate food substitutions to provide nutrients that may be missing from the diet. This is of particular concern for individuals with multiple food allergies.

Nutrition education should enable individuals with food allergy to:

- Define the allergen-free nutrition prescription
- List common foods that contain the allergen
- List foods that are allowed in an allergen-free nutrition prescription
- List nutrient-dense alternative foods that do not contain allergens
- Read a food label and state the risk involved in packaged foods with precautionary labeling.
- Be able to identify hidden sources of allergens
- Identify specialty companies that manufacture allergen-free foods in dedicated facilities
- Plan, shop for, and prepare healthy, allergen-free meals at home or in the homes of family and friends--this would include making substitutions in cooking as needed
- Select appropriate restaurants and interact with wait staff to choose meals that minimize the risk of allergen exposure
- Explain cross contamination risks and describe steps to take to minimize the risk
- Identify problem solving avoidance skills
- Describe symptoms of a food-induced allergic reaction and what should be done during a reaction
- Identify online resources for reliable medical information
- Locate and join food allergy support groups to share experiences with other food allergic families

The Food Allergen Labeling and Consumer Protection Act of 2004 (Title II of Public Law 108-282) was designed to help consumers identify immediately foods containing the eight major food allergens: milk, eggs, fish, Crustacean shellfish, tree nuts, peanuts, wheat, and soybeans with their usual or common name, *e.g.* "milk" "peanuts." This can help dietary managers and kitchen staff to immediately identify most foods with potential allergens; although, it should be noted that not all allergens are so identified. [3]

The presence of hidden allergens can be difficult to assess. If the dietary manager, licensed dietitian/nutritionist, or patient is in any doubt, they should contact the manufacturer.

Related foods, such as tree nuts, finned fish (the exception is canned tuna), and Crustaceans, may have common allergens and unless individuals have been tested and shown not to react to similar foods, all foods from related groups should be avoided. In exquisitely sensitive patients, it is also important not to cross contaminate cooking or serving utensils.

LABORATORY DATA INTERPRETATION

Blood Counts			
Test	**Normal**[1]	**Decreased**	**Increased**
WBC	$4.3-10^8$/L	Leukopenia (a decrease of WBC below 4,000/mm^3). Viral infections, some bacterial infections, overwhelming infection, chemotherapy, heavy metal intoxication, radiation, bone marrow depression, diuretics, cardiovascular drugs, HIV/AIDS, marrow-occupying diseases, iron deficiency anemia	Leukocytosis: acute infection, bacterial infection, leukemia, hemorrhage, trauma, tissue injury as occurs in surgery, cancer, after splenctomy, acute hemolysis.
RBC	M: $4.6-6.2\times10^6$ F: $4.2\times5.9\times10^6$	Anemia (nutritional and other), hemorrhage, systemic infection, leukemia, Lupus, Hodgkin's disease and other lymphomas	Erythrocytosis: primary: (polycythemia vera, erythrocytosis-erythremia); secondary: (renal, pulmonary, or cardiovascular disease; high altitude; tobacco; relative erythrocytosis: dehydration, stress, tobacco use, overuse of diuretics
Hematocrit	M: 45-52% F: 37-48%	Anemia (<30), blood loss, leukemia, hyperthyroidism, cirrhosis, over hydration , hemolysis, acute massive blood loss, cirrhosis	Severe dehydration,, polycythemia, shock
Hemoglobin	M: 13-18 g/dL F: 12.0-16.0 g/dL	Anemia, hyperthyroidism, cirrhosis, systemic diseases- (lupus, Hodgkin's, leukemia) prolonged dietary deficiencies, hemolytic reactions	With severe burns, CHF, polycythemia, COPD, dehydration,

[1]Laboratory values vary by individual labs and methodology used. These lab values were taken from: Hopkins T. Lab Notes: Nurse's Guide to Lab and Diagnositic Tests 3rd edition 2015. Philedelphia. F.A. Davis Company.
Abbreviations = WBC = white blood count, L = liter, HIV/AIDS = human immunodeficiency virus/acquired immunodeficiency syndrome, RBC = red blood cell, M = male, F = female, g = gram, dL = deciliter, CHF = congestive heart failure, COPD = chronic obstructive pulmonary disease.

	Clinical Chemistries		
Test	**Normal[1]**	**Decreased**	**Increased**
Sodium	136-145 mmol/L or 136-145 mEq/L	Hyponatremia: Addison's disease, severe burns, excessive fluid loss, edema, diuretics, nephritic syndrome, diabetic acidosis, dilutional from free water or hypotonic solutions, stomach suction with ice chips by mouth, CHF, diuretics	Dehydration, Conn's syndrome, primary aldosteronism, coma, Cushing's disease, diabetes insipidus, tracheobronchitis
Chloride	96-106 mmol/L or mEq/L	Severe vomiting, gastric secretion, chronic respiratory acidosis, burns, metabolic alkalosis, diabetes, Addison's disease, salt-losing diseases, overhydration, diuretic therapy	Dehydration, Cushing's syndrome, hyperventilation (respiratory alkalosis), metabolic disorders, hyperparathyroidism, renal tubular acidosis, diabetes insipidus
Potassium	3.5-5.0 mmol/L or mEq/L	Hypokalemia: Potassium depleting diuretics, GI losses-vomiting, diarrhea, fistulas, sweating alkalosis, malabsorption, alcohol abuse, chronic fever, hepatic disease w/ascites, hypercorticoidism Drugs-Excess licorice, steroids,salicylates,amphotericin.	Hyperkalemia: Addison's disease, acute renal failure, acidosis, tissue injury/damage, internal hemorrhage, uncontrolled DM, acute AIDS, hemolysis, malignant hyperpyrexia, cachexia, thrombocytosis, GI bleed, SLE, and sickle cell disease.
CO_2	23-30mEq/L	Severe diarrhea, starvation, acute renal failure, salicylate toxicity, diabetic acidosis, use of chlorothiazide diuretics	Severe vomiting, emphysema, aldosteronism, use of mercurial diuretics
Phosphorus/ Phosphate	2.5-4.5 mg/dL	Hyperparathroidism, GI losses, hypovitaminosis D, rickets, osteomalacia, hyperinsulinism, gout, overuse of PO_4 binders, Cushing's syndrome, salicylate poisoning, DM, alcoholism, refeeding syndrome	ESRD, Hypoparathyroidism, nephritis, diabetic acidosis hypocalcemia, bone tumors, Addison's disease, sickle cell anemia, acromegaly
Magnesium	1.6-2.2 mEq/L or 0.66-0.91 mmol/L	Magnesium containing antacids, pancreatitis, cirrhosis K+ depleting diuretics, hypothyroidism chronic diarrhea, alcoholism, ulcerative colitis, sweating, burns, malabsorption./malnutrition, multiple transfusions, gastric suction	Renal failure, diabetic acidosis, hypothyroidism, Addison's disease, dehydration, over use of Mg^{++} supplements or antacid, treatment of eclampsia, or alcohol withdrawal

Calcium	8.2-10.5 mg/dL	With hypoalbuminemia, (use corrected Ca^{++}) elevated phosphorus, chronic renal disease, uremia, diarrhea, Hypo parathyroidism, alkalosis, chronic rickets, sprue, osteomalacia, starvation, malabsorption, pancreatitis, hypomagnesemia, Vitamin D deficiency. Drugs including prolonged anti-convulsant therapy, steroid use, estrogens, insulin, phosphates, diuretics, fluorides, Mg^{++} salts, methicillin, laxatives, massive transfusion, alcoholism.	Hyperparathyroidism, multiple myeloma, cancers with or without bone involvement, Paget's disease of bone, immobilization, CRF, sarcoidosis adrenal insufficiency, long term use of thiazide diuretics, respiratory acidosis, milk-alkali syndrome, granulomatous disease , excessive use of vitamin D or calcium.
Calcium correction with hypoalbunemia For every 1mg/dL of albumin below 4 mg/dl, add 0.8 mg/dL to total calcium = [(4 - albumin) x 0.8] + calcium			

[1]Laboratory values vary by individual labs and methodology used. These lab values were taken from: Hopkins T. Lab Notes: Nurse's Guide to Lab and Diagnositic Tests 3rd edition 2015. Philedelphia. F.A. Davis Company.
Abbreviations = M = male, F = female, g = gram, dL = deciliter, CHF = congestive heart failure, AIDS = acquired immunodeficiency sydrome, mEqL = milliequivalent per liter, GI = gastrointestinal, DM = diabetes mellitus, SLE = systemic lupus erythematosus, ESRD = end stage renal disease, CRF = chronic renal failure, K = potassium, Ca = calcium, Mg = magnesium

Lipoprotein Tests and Creatine Phosphokinase

Test	Normal[1]	Decreased	Increased
Cholesterol	Desirable: <200 mg/dL Borderline: 200-239 mg/dL High: >240 mg/dL	Hypo-α-lipoproteinemia, severe hepatocellular disease, myeloproliferative diseases, hyperthyroidism, malabsorption/malnutrition, severe burns, inflammation, infection	Type II familial hypercholesterolemia, cholestasis, hepatocellular disease, nephritic syndrome, chronic renal failure, pancreatic cancer, poorly controlled diatetes, alcoholism, diet high in SFA, obesity
High-Density Lipoprotein Cholesterol	40-59 mg/dl ≥60 mg/dl is considered protective	Familial hypo-α-lipoproteinemia, triglyceridemia, poorly controlled diabetes, hepatocellular disease, cholestasis, chronic renal failure	Familial hyper-α-lipoproteinemia, chronic liver disease, long-term aerobic or vigorous exercise
Low-Density Lipoprotein Cholesterol	Desirable: <100 mg/dL Borderline: 130-159 mg/dL High risk: >160 mg/dL	Hypolipoproteinemia, Tangier disease, chronic anemias, severe hepatoceullular disease, Reye's syndrome, acute stress (burns, illness), inflammatory joint disease, chronic pulmonary disease	Diet high in SFA, hyperlipidemia secondary to hypothyroidism, nephritic syndrome, multiple myeloma, anorexia nervosa, diabetes, chronic renal failure, porphyria, premature CHD
Triglycerides	Desirable: <150 mg/dL Borderline:150-99mg/dL High: > 200-499 mg/dL Very High: ≥500 mg/dL	Congenital α-ß-lipoproteinemia, malnutrition/malabsorption, hyperthyroidism, COPD, brain infarction	Liver disease, nephrotic syndrome, alcoholism, hypothyroidism, myocardial infarction, hyperlipoproteinemias, alcohol abuse, pregnancy, contraceptive use, diabetes, chronic renal failure, and acute pancreatitis. Drugs, *e.g.* steroids, estrogens, cholestyramine, spironolactone, stress, high carbohydrate/fat diet. Non-fasting blood sample.
Creatine Phosphokinase (CPK)	M: 55-170 U/L F: 30-135 U/L		Myocardial infarction or cardiac trauma, acute CVA, ALS, vigorous exercise, hypothyroidism, muscular dystrophy, chronic alcoholism, pulmonary edema, hypokalemia

[1]Laboratory values vary by individual labs and methodology used. These lab values were taken from: Hopkins T. Lab Notes: Nurse's Guide to Lab and Diagnositic Tests 3rd edition 2015. Philedelphia. F.A. Davis Company. Abbreviations: M = male, F = female, mg = milligram, dL = deciliter, SFA = saturated fatty acids, COPD = chronic obstructive pulmonary disease, CHD = coronary heart disease, U = unit, L = liter; CVA = cerebrovascuar accident; ALS = Amyotrophic lateral sclerosis.

Labs Related to Glucose Metabolism			
Test	**Normal**[1]	**Decreased**	**Increased**
Fasting Blood Glucose	70-99 mg/dL	Hyperinsulinism- insulin overdose or oral hypoglycemic drugs, malnutrition, Addison's disease, adrenal cortical insuffiency, islet cell cancer, severe liver disease, glycogen storage disease, alcohol abuse, bacterial sepsis, hypothyroidism, vigorous exercise, pancreatitis, post gastrectomy, autonomic nervous system disorders, drugs/poisonings- *i.e.* alcohol, salicytes, phenformin, or antihistamines.	Diabetes mellitus, chronic hepatic dysfunction, Cushing's syndrome, pancreatitis, acute stress, Drugs--steroids, antihypertensives, estrogens, lithium, phenytoin, lasix, thiazides, thyroxine, caffeine, cyclosporine). Thiamine deficiency, hyperthyroidism, chronic liver disease, prolonged physical inactivity, or persistent uremia.
Glycosylated Hemoglobin (HbA$_{1c}$)	<5% of total hemoglobin (nondiabetic) 2.5-6% - well controlled diabetic >8% diabetes not well controlled	Hemolytic anemia, chronic blood loss, pregnancy, chronic renal failure	Poorly controlled diabetes, iron-deficiency anemia, spenectomy, alcohol toxicity, lead toxicity
C-Peptide (Fasting)	0.51-2.72 ng/mL	Facititious hypoglycemia, radical pancreatectomy, type 1 diabetes	Endogenous hyperinsulinism, oral hypoglycemic drugs, pancreas or ß-cell transplantation, type 2 diabetes.
Microalbuminuria/24 hour urine test	<30 mg/24 hours		Diabetes with early diabetic nephropathy, hypertension-heart disease, generalized vascular disease, preeclampsia.
[1]Laboratory values vary by individual labs and methodology used. These lab values were taken from: Hopkins T. Lab Notes: Nurse's Guide to Lab and Diagnositic Tests 3rd edition 2015. Philedelphia. F.A. Davis Company. Abbreviations: mg = milligram, dL = deciliter, ng = nanogram, mL = milliliter.			

End Products of Metabolism

Test	Normal[1]	Decreased	Increased
Blood Urea Nitrogen	10-20 mg/dL	Liver failure, acromegaly, malnutrition, celiac disease, nephritic syndrome, syndrome of inappropriate antidiuretic hormone	Impaired renal function caused by: CHF, salt and water depletion, shock, stress, acute MI; chronic renal disease, urinary tract obstruction, hemorrhage into GI tract, diabetes with ketoacidosis, excessive protein intake, anabolic steroid use
Creatinine	M: 0.6-1.2 mg/dL F: 0.5-1.1 mg/dL	Small stature, decreased muscle mass, advanced and severe liver disease, inadequate dietary protein, pregnancy	Acute and chronic renal functional impairment, lower urinary tract obstruction, CHF, chronic glomerulonephritis, muscle damage/disease, hyperthyroidism, starvation, acromegaly, gigantism, dehydration
Bilirubin	Total: 0.3-1.0 mg/dL Conjugated: 0.0-0.2 mg/dL		Total: Hemolytic or obstructive Jaundice, cirrhosis, destruction of RBC, cancer of pancreas or liver, hepatitis, biliary obstruction, reaction to drugs--chlorpromazine, pulmonary embolism, CHF. Conjugated: hemolytic anemias, trauma, cancer of the head of the pancreas, choledocholithiasis.
Ammonia	15-45 mcg/dL		Reye's syndrome, liver disease, cirrhosis, hepatic coma, GI hemorrhage, renal disease, inborn errors, TPN.
Uric acid	M: 4-8.5 mg/dL F: 2.8-7.3 mg/dL	With antigout meds, after intake of ACTH and aspirin, Wilson's Disease, Fanconi's disease, Xanthinuria, some neoplasms (*i.e.* Hodgkins, Myeloma, Bronchogenic Cancers). Healthy adults are often below references.	Gout, nephrosis, renal failure, neoplasms, leukemia, toxemia of pregnancy, psoriasis, sarcoidosis, alcohol consumption, obese patient on reduction diet. Drugs-diuretics, catecholamines, ethambutol, pyrazinamide, salicylates, and nicotinic acid

[1]Laboratory values vary by individual labs and methodology used. These lab values were taken from:
Hopkins T. Lab Notes: Nurse's Guide to Lab and Diagnositic Tests 3rd edition 2015. Philedelphia. F.A. Davis Company.
Abbreviations: M = male, F = female, g = gram, dL = deciliter, CHF = congestive heart failure, GI = gastrointestinal, RBC = red blood cells, TPN = total parenteral nutrition, ACTH = Adrenocorticotropic hormone.

Enzyme Tests			
Test	**Normal**[1]	**Decreased**	**Increased**
Aspartate Transaminase (AST) (aka serum glutamic-oxaloacetic transaminase [SGOT])	0-35 U/L	Azotemia, chronic renal dialysis, vitamin B6 deficiency	Acute and chronic hepatitis, active cirrhosis, infectious mononucleosis, hepatic necrosis and metastasis, primary and metastatic carcinoma, alcoholic hepatitis, MI, hypothyroidism, trauma, Duchene's muscular dystrophy, mushroom poisoning, shock, hemolytic anemia, exhaustion, heat stroke
Alanine Aminotransferase (ALT) (aka serum glutamic-pyruvic transaminase ([SGPT])	M: 10-35 U/L		Hepatocellular disease, alcoholic chirrhosis, metastatic liver tumor, obstructive jaundice, infectious mononucleosis, pancreatitis, severe burns, shock
Alkaline phosphatase (ALP)	42-136 U/L	Hypophosphatasia, malnutrition, hypothyroidism, pernicious and severe anemias, scurvy, Mg and Zn deficiency, Vitamin D excess, milk-alkali syndrome, cretinism, dwarfism, kwashiorkor, deposition of radioactive materials in bone	Increased osteoblastic activity-osteomalacia, hyperparathyroidism, hepatobiliary disease, rickets, Vitamin D deficiency, osteogenic imperfecta, Paget's disease, metastatic bone disease, bone growth (children/pregnancy), ulcerative colitis, chronic renal failure, CHF
Lactic dehydrogenate (LDH/LD)	100-190 U/L LDH_1: 17-27% LDH_2: 27-37% LDH_3: 18-25% LDH_4: 3-8% LDH_5: 0-5%	Not clinically significant	LDH_1: MI, megaloblastic anemia, hemolytic anemia, muscular dystrophy. LDH_2: MI, granulocytic leukemia, pancreatitis, megaloblastic anemia, hemolytic anemia, muscular dystrophy. LDH_3: Granulocytic leukemia, pancreatitis. LDH_4: Pulmonary infarction, CHF, viral and toxic hepatitis. LDH_5: Pulmonary infarction, CHF, viral and toxic hepatitis.
Amylase	60-160 Somogyi U/dL	Pancreatic Insufficiency, hepatitis, severe liver disease, advanced cystic fibrosis, pancreatectomy	Pancreatic disorders (*e.g.* pancreatitis, alcoholic and non-alcoholic, pancreatic carcinoma); partial gastrectomy, appendicitis, peritonitis, perforated peptic ulcer, cerebral trauma, ruptured tubal pregnancy, ruptured aortic aneurysm.
Lipase	0-60 U/L		Pancreatic disorders (*e.g.* pancreatitis, alcoholic and non-alcoholic, pancreatic carcinoma); cholecystitis, hemodialysis, strangulated bowel, peritonitis, primary biliary cirrhosis, chronic renal failure

[1]Laboratory values vary by individual labs and methodology used. These lab values were taken from: Hopkins T. Lab Notes: Nurse's Guide to Lab and Diagnositic Tests 3rd edition 2015. Philedelphia. F.A. Davis Company.Abbreviations: M = male, F = female, U = unit, L = liter, MI = myocardial infarction, CHF = congestive heart failure.

Assessment of Protein Status			
Test	**Normal[1]**	**Decreased**	**Increased**
Albumin	3.5-5 gm/dL	Acute and chronic inflammation, cirrhosis, liver disease, alcoholism, nephritic syndrome, inflammatory bowel disease, burns, severe skin disease, heart failure, starvation, malnutrition, malabsorption, anorexia, Cushing's syndrome, overhydration; Stress/Trauma	Dehydration, corticosteroid therapy, administration of exogenous albumin
Prealbumin	20-40 mg/dL	Acute and chronic inflammation, cirrhosis, liver disease, alcoholism, nephritic syndrome, inflammatory bowel disease, burns, severe skin disease, heart failure, starvation, malnutrition, malabsorption, anorexia, overhydration. Stress/Trauma	Dehydration
Transferrin	220-430 mg/dL	Microcytic anemia of chronic disease, protein deficiency or loss from burns, malnutrition, chronic infection, acute liver disease, nephrosis, hereditary atransferrinemia, hemochromatoris	Iron deficiency anemia, pregnancy, estrogen therapy
Retinol-binding protein	2.6-7.6 mg/dL[2]	Uncomplicated protein-energy malnutrition, compromised retinol status	

[1]Laboratory values vary by individual labs and methodology used. These lab values were taken from:
Hopkins T. Lab Notes: Nurse's Guide to Lab and Diagnositic Tests 3rd edition 2015. Philedelphia. F.A. Davis Company.
[2]Mahan LK, Escott-Stump S. Krause's Food & Nutrition Therapy. 2015. St. Louis, MO. Saunders Elsevier.
Abbreviations: gm = gram, dL = deciliter, mg = milligram

Nitrogen Balance Calculations

Nitrogen balance = nitrogen intake - nitrogen losses

Nitrogen intake = protein intake/6.25

Nitrogen losses = urinary urea nitrogen (UUN) + non-urea urinary nitrogen (1-2 g) + fecal nitrogen (1-2 g) + miscellaneous losses from skin and sweat (~1g or 0.1-0.5 g/m^2)

Nitrogen balance (gm) = (protein intake in gm) - (UUN excretion in gm + 3-5 gm) x 6.25 of nitrogen/gm of protein.

DRUG-NUTRIENT INTERACTIONS

RECOMMENDATIONS

The identification of the management of certain drugs with potential drug-nutrient interaction is beneficial in the nutritional management of patients using these drugs. Methods of monitoring drug interactions must be made part of the total patient care plan. Physician, pharmacists, nurses and dietitians participate in both the planning and review process. The main concern of the dietitian is how the drug-nutrient action affects the patient's sense of taste and smell, swallowing, waste elimination, contribution to a lessened total dietary intake that results in risk factors for malnutrition, or increase or decrease in drug bioavailability.

Drugs that may contribute to nutrient alterations include, but are not limited to the following:

1. Cardiac Glycosides
2. Antihypertensives
3. Antianginal
4. Diuretics
5. Anti-inflammatory agents
6. Antacids (antacid overuse)
7. Anti-GERD or gastritis agents
8. Laxatives (laxative overuse)
9. Psychotropic drugs
10. Anti-Coagulants
11. Anti-Convulsants
12. Anti-Lipomics

In addition, the Federal Omnibus Budget Reconciliation Act guidelines outline 10 classes of drugs that contribute to nutritional deficiencies: Antacids, Anti-inflammatory, Anticonvulsants, Antineoplastics, Antiarrhythmics, Diuretics, Laxatives, Oral Hypoglycemics, Phenothiazines, Psychotropics

Selected drugs under these classifications are listed by generic and brand name along with nutritional considerations, possible gastrointestinal effects and recommended actions.

Medications With Potential Drug – Nutrient Interactions			
Medication	**Possible Dietary Significance**	**Possible Laboratory Significance**	**Recommended Dietary Actions**
CARDIOGLYCOSIDES Antiarhythmic/Stimulants Dioxin (Lanoxin, Lanoxicaps, Crystodigin)	Anorexia leading to reduced intake and weight loss; nausea/vomiting	Hypokalemia with potassium wasting diuretics ↑ Serum calcium ↓ Serum magnesium Potential for drug toxicity with hypoalbuminemia <3.0 gm/dl	Monitor electrolytes Maintain diet ↑ in potassium Avoid natural licorice and herbal teas
ANTIHYPERTENSIVES Captopril (Capoten) Propranolol (Inderal) Felodipine (Plendil) Calan (Verapamil)	Dry mouth, taste changes nausea/vomiting, diarrhea	↑ Serum glucose ↑ Serum K ↓ Serum Na ↑ BUN, ↑ creatinine	Monitor use of potassium supplements and salt substitutes. Avoid use of herbs with hypertensive properties.[1] Do not take with grapefruit or grapefruit juice
ANTIANGINAL Diltlazemn (Cardizem) Nifedipene (Procadia)	Nausea, dry mouth, altered taste, anorexia Constipation May see weight gain due to edema		Low sodium diet may be needed with edema Avoid use of herbs with hypertensive properties.[1] Do not take with grapefruit or grapefruit juice
DIURETICS A. Potassium-sparing Spironolactone (Aldactone) Traimeterene (Dyrenium) B. Potassium-wasting Bumetanide (Bumex) HCTZ (Esidrex, Hydrodiuril, Oretic, Dyazide, Maxide)	Anorexia, diarrhea, GI cramps	↑ Serum K ↓ Serum Na ↑ BUN, creatinine May ↑ Serum glucose	Monitor potassium Avoid natural licorice and salt substitutes. Low sodium diet may also be needed . Avoid use of herbs with hypertensive properties.[1]
Acetazolamde (Diamox) Chlorothiazide (Diuril) Furosemide (Lasix) Ethacrynic Acid (Edecrin) Metolazone (Diulo, Zaroxolyn)	GI irritation, anorexia, nausea/vomiting, diarrhea, dry mouth	↑ Serum glucose ↓ Serum Na ↓ Serum K ↑ BUN, ↑ creatinine ↓ Serum calcium (Lasix, Bumex, Edecrin)	Monitor electrolytes. Avoid natural licorice. Maintain high potassium diet if not on potassium supplement. Monitor glucose. Avoid use of herbs with hypertensive properties.[1]
[1]Herbs with hypertensive properties include: Bayberry, Blue Cohosh, Cayenne, Ephedra (removed from market), Ginger, Ginseng (American), Kola, Natural Licorice.			

Medication	Possible Dietary Significance	Possible Laboratory Significance	Recommended Dietary Actions
ANTI-INFLAMMATORY AGENTS			
A. Corticosteroids Prednisolone Prednisone (Deltasone, Orasone) Hydrocortisone (Corter) Dexamethasone (Decadron Hexadrol) Betamethasone (Nalfon)	GI distress, GI inflammation/bleeding ↑ appetite ↑ weight Prolonged use can ↓ absorption of Ca and P and ultimately affect bone density. Prolonged use can also alter CHO and protein metabolism. Prolonged use can affect following vitamin status: Vitamin A, C, D, folate, pyridoxine	↑ Serum cholesterol ↑ Serum triglycerides ↑ Serum sodium ↓ Serum calcium ↓ Serum zinc ↓ bioavailability	Monitor electrolytes. May need foods ↑ in potassium Vitamin A, C, D, folate, calcium phosphorus. May need low sodium diet if edema occurs. Monitor glucose levels. Avoid antacids
B. Antiarthritic/NSAID Analgesic Naproxen (Naprosyn, Anaprox) Ketorolactromethamine (Toradol) Ibuprofen (Advil, Medipren, Motrin, Nupren, Rufolin) Indomethacin (Indocen) Salsalate (Disalcid) Sulendac (Clinoril) Piroxicam (Feldene) Dfunisal (Dolobid)	GI distress, GI inflammation/bleeding, diarrhea, stomatitis, dry mouth, ↓ appetite	↑ BUN ↑ Creatinine ↑ Serum potassium ↓ Serum glucose	Monitor glucose level Avoid use of herbs with anticoagulant/antiplatelet properties[1]
C. Analgesic/NSAID, Antipyretic Acetylsalicylic acid (Aspirin, Anacin, Ascriptin, Bufferin, Ecotrin, Empiren) Acetaminophen (Anacin 3, Datril, Panadol, Tempra, Tylenol)	GI distress can be minimized if taken with food. Can cause GI bleeding, nausea/vomiting. May contribute to iron deficiency anemia. Fewer incidences of GI distress and GI bleeding. Can cause hemolytic anemia.	↓ Serum folate ↓ Serum Vitamin C	Insure adequate fluids. Increase foods high in Vitamin C and folic acid. Insure adequate fluids. Avoid use of herbs with anticoagulant/antiplatelet properties.[1]

[1]Herbs with anticoagulant/antiplatelet properties include: Alfalfa, Anise, Bilberry, Bladderwrack, Bromelain, Cat's Claw, Celery, Coleus, Cordyceps, Dong, Quai, Evening Primrose Oil, Fenugreek, Feverfew, Garlic, Ginger, Ginkgo Biloba, Ginseng (American, Panax, or Siberian), Grape Seed, GreenTea, Guggul, Horse Chestnut Seed, Horseradish, Natural Licorice, Prickly Ash, Red Clover, Reishi, SAMe, Sweet Clover, Turmeric, White Willow.

Medication	Possible Dietary Significance	Possible Laboratory Significance	Recommended Dietary Actions
ANTACIDS Aluminum carbonate (Basalgel) Aluminum hydroxide (Alucapo, Alternagel, Amphogel Dialume) Aluminum hydroxide and Magnesium hydroxide (Gelusil, Maalox, Maalox Plus, Mylanta) Calcium carbonate (Tums, Rolaids)	With large doses or prolonged use: anorexia, constipation, diarrhea, chalky dry mouth. Can inactivate thiamin. Decreases absorption of phosphorus, iron and Vitamin A. May cause osteomalacia, osteoporosis. Significant source of calcium if not taken with foods high in phytic acid. Anorexia, constipation. Decreases absorption of iron, phosphorus, Vitamin A. Can cause dry chalky mouth.	↑ Serum alkaline phosphotase ↓ Serum phosphorus ↑ Serum aluminum Aluminum hydroxide and Magnesium hydroxide: ↑ Serum Magnesium Calcium Carbonate: ↑ Serum calcium ↓ Serum phosphorus	Insure adequate hydration. If used for phosphate binding therapy take with water or juice. If used as antacid, take 1-3 hours after meals. Take with meals as calcium supplement or phosphate binder. Take 1-3 hours after meals as antacids.
Anti-GERD or gastritis AGENTS Cimetidene (Tagamet); Ranitidine (Zantac); Sucralfate (Carafate)	Constipation, diarrhea, nausea	↑ Creatinine ↓ Serum B12	Limit caffeine

Medication	Possible Dietary Significance	Possible Laboratory Significance	Recommended Dietary Actions
LAXATIVES Milk of Magnesia (MOM) Mineral Oil	Nausea, diarrhea May decrease absorption of fat soluble vitamins, calcium, phosphorus. With prolonged use: weight loss, anorexia		Increase fluids. Increase fluids, fiber.
Bisacodyl (Dulcolax)	Decreases intestinal absorption of glucose. With prolonged use: decreases intestinal absorption of amino acids, weight loss	Long term use: ↑ Serum calcium ↓ Serum potassium	Increase fluids, fiber
Lactulose (Cephulac, Chr onulac)	Diarrhea, nausea		Increase fluids. Do not use with lactose or galactose free diet
Docusate Sodium (Colace, Dialose) Docusate Sodium (Surfak)	Alters intestinal absorption of water and electrolytes. Can cause throat irritation, bitter after taste, nausea, diarrhea	↑ Serum glucose ↓ Serum potassium	Increase fluids, fiber.

Phenolphtalein (Modane, Correctal, Ex-Lax)	Diarrhea, cramping, nausea Long term: malabsorption and steatorrhea, osteomalacia	Long term use: ↓ Serum potassium ↓ Serum sodium ↓ Serum calcium ↑ Serum glucose	Increase fluids, fiber.
Psylluem, hydrophilic mucilloid (Fiberall, Metamucil, Perdiem)	May decrease appetite, cause abdominal cramping, bloating	↓ Serum cholesterol ↓ Serum LDL	Increase fluid. Use with caution in diabetes.
Senna (Senokot)	Long term use: fluid and electrolyte imbalance	↑ Serum glucose ↓ Serum potassium ↓ Serum calcium	

Medication	Possible Dietary Significance	Possible Laboratory Significance	Recommended Dietary Actions
PSYCHOTROPICS A. Anti-Psychotics Haloperidol (Haldol)	Anorexia, decreased thirst, dehydration, dry mouth, dyspepsia, constipation		
Loxapen (Loxitane)	Dry mouth, nausea/vomiting, constipation		
Molendone (Moban)	Anorexia, weight loss, dry mouth, nausea, constipation		Monitor diabetes
Thiothixene (Navene) Prochlorperazine (Compazine)	Increase appetite, increases weight. Can cause dry mouth, constipation, nausea/vomiting.		May need to monitor calories. Monitor diabetes
Chlorpromazine (Thorazine) Thioridazine (Mellaril)	Interferes with riboflavin metabolism. Increases appetite, increases weight. Dry mouth, nausea/vomiting, constipation		Encourage foods high in riboflavin (dairy products, dark leafy vegetables, enriched cereals). May need to reduce calories.
B. Anti-Depressants Bupropion (Wellbutrin)	Anorexia, weight loss, dry mouth, constipation.		Limit caffeine.
Doxepin (Sinequan)	Increase appetite, weight		Monitor diabetes Avoid St. Johns Wort
Fluoxetene (Prozac)	Cause dry mouth, metallic sour after taste, epegastric distress, constipation.		Tryptophan supplement enhances side effects.
Paroxetine (Paxil)	Anorexia, weight loss, dry mouth, taste changes, dyspepsia, constipation		Monitor diabetes.
C. Monoamine Oxidase Inhibitors (MAOI) (Antidepressants) Tranylcypromine Sulfate (Parnate) Phenelzene Sulfate (Nordil, Marpean)	Increase appetite, weight gain. Can cause dry mouth, nausea, constipation. Alters vitamin B_6 metabolism May need vitamin B_6 supplement. Can cause dry mouth, nausea, or constipation		Monitor diabetes. Limit caffeine. Avoid trypotophan supplement. Avoid food high in pressor amines: aged cheese, meats, liver, sausage, pickled herring, fava beans, bananas, avocados, fermented bean curds, alcohol, alcohol-free beer.

Medication	Possible Dietary Significance	Possible Laboratory Significance	Recommended Dietary Actions
ANTI-COAGULANTS Warfarin (Coumadin)	Can cause nausea/vomiting or diarrhea. Drug effects increased with albumin <3.0 gm/dl.	Coumadin has a narrow therapeutic range and levels need to be monitored.	Do not vary amount of meat, dairy products and green leafy vegetables eaten on a given day. These foods are high in Vitamin K and can affect blood clotting measurements. Avoid use of herbs with anticoagulant/antiplatelet properties.[1]
ANTI-CONVULSANTS Phenobarbital Phenytoin (Dilantin)	Increases metabolism of Vitamin D and Vitamin K. Long term use can alter B_{12} and folic acid status. Can cause nausea, vomiting, gum hyperplasia, dry mouth.	↓ Serum folate ↓ Serum B_{12} ↑ Serum cholesterol ↓ Serum calcium ↓ Serum magnesium ↓ Serum phosphorus	Increase Vitamin D and calcium intake. Limit caffeine. Long term: may need folic acid and B_{12} supplements. Avoid use of herbs with anticoagulant/antiplatelet properties.[1]
Carbamazipene (Tegretol)	Can cause anorexia, dry mouth, nausea/vomiting, diarrhea	↑ BUN ↓ Serum calcium ↑ Serum cholesterol	Increase Vitamin D and calcium intake.

[1]Herbs with anticoagulant/antiplatelet properties include: Alfalfa, Anise, Bilberry, Bladderwrack, Bromelain, Cat's Claw, Celery, Coleus, Cordyceps, Dong, Quai, Evening Primrose Oil, Fenugreek, Feverfew, Garlic, Ginger, Ginkgo Biloba, Ginseng (American, Panax, or Siberian), Grape Seed, Green Tea, Guggul, Horse Chestnut Seed, Horseradish, Natural Licorice, Prickly Ash, Red Clover, Reishi, SAMe, Sweet Clover, Turmeric, White Willow.

Medication	Possible Dietary Significance	Possible Laboratory Significance	Recommended Dietary Actions
ANTI-LIPOMICS Cholestyramine (Questram)	May decrease absorption of calcium, fat soluble vitamins, folic acid, glucose. May cause anorexia, nausea/vomiting, constipation or diarrhea.	↓ Serum cholesterol ↓ Serum calcium ↓ Serum potassium ↓ Serum sodium ↓ Serum folate	Diet low in saturated fatty acids and cholesterol recommended to enhance drug results. Fat soluble and folic acid supplements recommended.
Gemfibrozil (Lobid)	May cause dyspepsia and diarrhea.	↓ Serum cholesterol ↑ Serum glucose ↑ Serum HDL ↓ Serum LDL	Monitor diabetes. Diet low in saturated fatty acids, with reduced calories recommended if weight loss is desired.
Lovastaten (Mevacor)	May cause nausea, dyspepsia and constipation	↓ Serum cholesterol ↓ Serum LDL, VLDL ↑ Serum HDL	Diet low in saturated fatty acids and cholesterol recommended to enhance drug results. Do not take with Niacin supplements.
Coleslipol (colestid)	May decrease absorption of fat soluble vitamins including Vitamin K. Can cause abdominal pain and bloating, anorexia, constipation.	↓ Serum LDL ↓ Serum cholesterol ↓ Serum Vitamin K ↓ Serum potassium ↓ Serum sodium	Diet low in saturated fatty acids and cholesterol recommended to enhance drug results. Increase fluids and fiber in diet. Vitamins A, D and K supplements recommended.

168

Common HIV/ AIDS Medications and their diet-nutrient Interactions				
Class of Drug	**Drug Name**	**Side Effects**	**Administration Recommendations**	**Nutrient Interactions to Avoid**
Protease Inhibitor	Amprenavir	NVD, abdominal pain, taste change, lipid alterations, glucose intolerance	Take separately from antacids and Ca and Mg supplements	Contraindications associated with taking with high-fat meal , ethanol, garlic, garlic St. John's Wort.[18, 19]
	Atazanavir	NVD, taste change, glucose intolerance, lipo-dystrophy	Take with food; take 2 hours before or 1 hour after taking Ca or Mg supplements or antacids	Contraindications associated with St. John's Wort.
	Darunavir	NVD, abdominal pain, lipid alterations, glucose intolerance, lipo-dystrophy	Take with food	Contraindications associated with ethanol.
	Indinavir	NVD, anorexia, abdominal pain, lipo-dystrophy,	Take on an empty stomach, or with a light, low-fat snack	Contraindications associated with grapefruit juice and St. John's Wort.
	Lopinavir	NVD, abdominal pain, lipid alterations, glucose intolerance, lipo-dystrophy	Take with food; high fat increases drug level	Contraindications associated with St. John's Wort.
	Nelfinavir	NV, abdominal pain	No available recommendations	Contraindications associated with St. John's Wort.
	Ritonavir	NVD, abdominal pain, lipo-dystrophy	Take with food	Contraindications associated with ethanol and St. John's Wort.

	Saquinavir	NVD, abdominal pain, taste change, lipid alterations, glucose intolerance	Take with food	Contraindications associated with grapefruit and associated citrus, garlic and St. John's Wort.
	Tipranavir	NVD, anorexia, lipid alterations, glucose intolerance, lipo-dystrophy	Take with a full meal, preferable high fat	Contraindications associated with St. John's Wort.
Nucleoside Reverse Transcriptase Inhibitors	Abacavir	NVD, anorexia, abdominal pain	No available recommendations	Contraindications associated with ethanol.
	Didanosine	NVD, anorexia, abdominal pain, taste change, lipid alterations	Take without food half hour before or 1 hour after eating	Contraindications associated with ethanol, and Mg supplement.
	Emtricitabine	NVD, anorexia, lipid alterations	No available recommendations	Contraindications associated with ethanol.
	Zalcitabine	NVD, anorexia, abdominal pain	Take on an empty stomach, 1 hr pre, 2 hr post	Contraindications associated with ethanol.
	Lamivudine	NVD, anorexia, abdominal pain	Take with food	No contraindications found.
	Stavudine	NVD, anorexia, abdominal pain, lipid alterations, lipo-dystrophy	No available recommendations	No contraindications found.
Non-Nucleoside Reverse Transcriptase Inhibitors	Delavirdine	NVD, anorexia	Take with acidic beverage, separate from antacids 1hr	Contraindications associated with ethanol, grapefruit and associated citrus, and St. John's Wort.
	Efavirenz	NVD, anorexia, abdominal pain,	No available recommendations	Contraindications associated with taking with high fat meal and

		lipid alterations		St. John's Wort.
	Etravirine	NVD, anorexia, abdominal pain, lipo-dystrophy	Take after a meal	No contraindications found.
	Nevirapine	NVD, anorexia, abdominal pain, glucose intolerance	No available recommendations	Contraindications associated with St. John's Wort.
	Tenofovir	NVD, anorexia, abdominal pain, lipo-dystrophy	High fat meal increases bioavailability	No contraindications found.
Fusion Inhibitor	Zidovudine	NV, anorexia	Avoid a high fat meal	No contraindications found.
Integrase Inhibitor	Enfuvirtide	Anorexia, taste change, lipid alterations	No available recommendations	Contraindications associated with St. John's Wort.
Entry Inhibitor	Raltegravir	NVD, anorexia, abdominal pain, lipo-dystrophy	No available recommendations	Contraindications associated with ethanol.
	Maraviroc	NVD, anorexia, abdominal pain	No available recommendations	Contraindications associated with ethanol and St. John's Wort.

SELECTED FOOD SOURCES

Source of all tables with food sources of nutrients: United States Department of Agriculture Agricultural Research Service Database

Selected Food Sources
of Calcium

Food	Serving Size	Calcium (mg)/serving
Yogurt, low fat with fruit	1cup	345
Rhubarb, cooked	½ cup	318
Spinach frozen, cooked	1 cup	291
Milk, 2%	1 cup	286
Buttermilk, reduced fat	1 cup	284
Milk, whole	1cup	276
Cottage, cheese, 2%	1 cup	206
Cheese, cheddar	1 oz	204
Salmon, canned with bones	3 ½ oz	181
Tofu, regular	¼ block	163
Egg custard	½ cup	151
Vanilla Ice cream	½ cup	125
Ice-cream, softserve	½ cup	113
Turnip Greens	½ cup	105
Almonds	1 oz	70
Baked beans, white	½ cup	64
Broccoli, cooked from fresh	1 cup	62
Okra, boiled	½ cup	62
Frankfurter , turkey	1	58
Orange	1	52
Halibut, baked	medium	51
Kale, cooked	3 oz	47
Bread, whole wheat	½ cup	20
Banana	1 slice	7
Ground beef, lean	1 medium 3 oz	4

172

SELECTED FOOD SOURCES OF VITAMIN A*

HIGH		MEDIUM	
More than 4000 IU	**Serving Size**	**More than 300 IU**	**Serving Size**
Liver, Calf, cooked	3 oz.	Butter or Margarine	1 T
Cantaloupe	1 cup	Cheese (most)	1 oz.
Mango, raw	½ medium	Ice Cream	½ cup
Butternut Squash	½ cup	Milk	1 cup
Carrots, raw or cooked	½ cup	Tangerine	½ cup
Cooked Greens (collards, mustard, turnip)	½ cup	Asparagus	½ cup
		Green Beans	½ cup
Pumpkin, canned	2 T	Brussels Sprouts	½ cup
Cooked Spinach	½ cup	Corn	4 in ear
Sweet Potato, small, baked	1	Green Peas	½ cup
		Summer Squash, raw or cooked Avocado	½ cup
			½ medium
		Fruit Cocktail	½ cup
		Pink Grapefruit	½ medium
More than 2000 IU	**Serving Size**	**Orange Juice, canned or fresh**	**1 cup**
Apricots	3 medium	Prunes	3
Papaya	½ medium	Peach, raw	1 medium
Broccoli, raw or cooked	1 large stalk	Watermelon	1 cup
Acorn Squash	½ medium	Tomatoes, raw or canned	1 small

SELECTED FOOD SOURCES OF VITAMIN C

Food	Serving Size	Vitamin C (mg)/serving
Peppers, sweet, yellow	½ cup	171
Peppers, sweet, red	½ cup	95
Kiwi fruit	½ cup	82
Orange juice, raw	½ cup	62
Peppers, sweet, green	½ cup	60
Strawberries	½ cup	49
Orange juice, diluted from concentrate	½ cup	48
Oranges	½ cup	48
Grapefruit juice, white raw	½ cup	47
Mandarin oranges, canned	½ cup	43
Grapefruit	½ cup	38
Mandarin oranges, fresh	½ cup	36
Cantaloupe	½ cup	33

Broccoli, fresh, cooked, chopped	½ cup	31
Kale	½ cup	27
Mango	½ cup	23
Tomato Juice	½ cup	22
Tomato	½ cup	11
Potatoes	½ cup	10

SELECTED FOOD SOURCES OF FIBER

Food	Serving Size	Fiber (g)/serving
100% ready-to-eat bran cereal	½ cup	8.8
Red kidney beans	½ cup	8.2
Split peas, cooked	½ cup	8.0
Lentils, cooked	½ cup	7.8
Black beans, cooked	½ cup	7.5
Globe artichoke	1	6.5
Sweet potato, cooked with skin	1 medium	4.8
Raspberries, red	½ cup	4.0
Mixed vegetables	½ cup	4.0
Green beans, cooked	1 cup	4.0
Prunes	½ cup	3.8
Potato, baked with skin	1 medium	3.8
Brown rice, cooked	1 cup	3.5
Spinach	½ cup	3.5
Apple, raw with skin	1 medium	3.3
Almonds	1 oz	3.3
Banana	1 medium	3.1
Orange	1 medium	3.1
Broccoli	½ cup	2.8
Peas	½ cup	2.5
Corn	½ cup	2.3
Whole-wheat bread	1 slice	1.9

SELECTED FOOD SOURCES OF IRON

Food	Serving Size	Iron (mg)
Fortified ready-to-eat cereal	1cup	1-22
Clams, canned	3oz	23.7
Rice, white enriched	1 cup	9.73
Baked beans	1 cup	8.2
Braunschweiger	2 slices	6.35
Oysters, cooked	3 oz	5.9
Liver, Beef fried	3 oz	5.24
Spinach, cooked	1 cup	6.43
Corn dog	1	6.18
Blueberries, frozen	½ cup	4.5
Refried Beans	1 cup	4.18
Potato skin	1	4.08
Ground beef, lean	3 oz	1.8
Apricots, dried	½ cup	1.73
Molasses	1 T	0.94
Raisins	1 oz	0.53
Salmon	3 oz	0.47

Cast iron cookware may contribute slightly to the iron content of food, especially when cooking acid food. The absorption of non-heme iron is increased by concomitant intake of food high in vitamin C

SELECTED FOOD SOURCES OF PURINE

100-1000 mg of Purine Nitrogen/100g food (HIGH)		9 to 100 mg of Purine Nitrogen/100 g food (MODERATE)		Negligible Purine Content (LOW)	
Foods in this group should be admitted from the diets of patients with gout		One serving (2-3 oz) of meat, fist, or fowl, or 1 ½ cup serving of vegetables is allowed each day		Food may be used with impunity	
Anchovies	Meat extracts	Fish	Asparagus	Bread, white	Fruit
Bouillon	Mincemeat	Poultry	Beans, dried	Butter	Gelatin
Brains	Mussels	Meat	Cauliflower	Cake	desserts
Broth	Partridge	Shellfish	Lentils	Cookies	Herbs
Consommé	Roe		Mushrooms	Cereal	Ice Cream
Goose	Sardines		Oatmeal	beverage	Milk
Gravy	Scallops		Peas, dried	Cereals	Macaroni
Heart	Sweetbreads		Spinach	Cheese	products
Herring	Yeast		Wheat germ	Chocolate	Noodles
Kidney	(brewers and		and bran	Coffee	Nuts

Mackerel	bakers--supplements)			Condiments Cornbread Crackers Cream Custard Eggs Fats Vegetables (over than those in group 2)	Oil Olives Pickles Popcorn Puddings Relishes Rice Slat Sugar and Sweets Tea Vinegar White Sauce

Sodium and Potassium Content of Selected Foods				
Food	Amount	Kcals	Sodium (mg)	Potassium (mg)
Beverages	12 oz	144	4	0
Coca-Cola	12 oz	160	2	0
Pepsi-Cola	12 oz	1	63	30
Pepsi-Cola sugar free	12 oz	142	46	0
Sprite	12 oz	120	22	40
Hawaiian Punch	8 oz	133	10	50
Lemonade from Frozen Concentrate	1 cup	102	13	33
Lemonade Flavored Drink (from dry mix)	1 tsp.	4	1	64
Coffee-instant	powder	2	1	46
Tea-instant powder	1 tsp.			
Condiments, Spreads, Dressings				
Barbecue sauce	1 Tbsp.	12	127	27
Mustard, yellow	1 tsp.	4	63	7
Pickles, cucumber dill	1 medium	7	928	130
Soy sauce	1 Tbsp.	6	822	22
Worcestershire sauce	1 Tbsp.	11	234	40
Butter (salted)	1 tsp.	36	41	1
Margarine	1 tsp.	34	37	4
French dressing	1 Tbsp.	22	128	13
Italian dressing	1 Tbsp.	69	116	2
Mayonnaise-type dressing	1 Tbsp.	57	105	1
Thousand Island dressing	1 Tbsp.	59	109	18
Desserts, Candies And Sweets				
Cookie - chocolate chip	2	99	84	28
Cookie - oatmeal (commercial)	2	130	90	35
Custard, vanilla	½ cup	143	83	176

Doughnut - raised, yeast	1 average	105	139	27
Gelatin dessert, all 3 flavors	½ cup	80	95	0
Ice Cream - vanilla	½ cup	134	58	128
Pudding - vanilla	½ cup	162	190	191
Sherbet, orange	½ cup	97	44	99
Milk Chocolate Bar (Hershey)	1	254	35	193
Lifesavers	5 pieces	46	5	0
M&M's - regular	1 pkg.	172	34	137
Marshmallows	1 average	19	2	0
Baby Ruth	1 bar	260	120	120
Honey	1 Tbsp.	64	1	11
Jelly - all varieties	1 Tbsp.	49	3	14
Molasses, light	1 Tbsp.	50	3	183
Sugar - dark brown	1 Tbsp.	34	3	31
Sugar - white granular	½ cup	385	1	3
Syrup - maple	5 Tbsp.	250	10	176
Appetizers & Snack Foods	1 oz.	167	3	219
Almonds, not salted	1 oz.	163	4	160
Cashew Nuts, roasted	1 Tbsp.	24	84	26
Dip - French onion	1 oz.	33	164	87
Dip - bean	⅔ oz.	90	183	160
Peanuts, roasted and salted	12 halves	95	0	55
Pecans, shelled	½ oz.	83	2	104
Almonds - dried, unblanched	½ oz.	82	2	80
Breads and Cereals				
All-Bran cereal	⅓ cup	71	320	350
Bran Flakes (40%)	¾ cup	93	264	180
Cheerios	¾ cup	75	174	63
Cornflakes	¾ cup	75	226	24
Puffed Wheat	¾ cup	37	1	37
Shredded Wheat	1 biscuit	83	0	77
Oatmeal - cooked, without salt	¾ cup	108	1	99
Rice - white - cooked without salt	½ cup	111	4	29
Cream of Wheat - regular - cooked	¾ cup	100	2	33
Malt-o-meal - cooked without salt	¾ cup	92	2	35
Graham crackers	2 crackers	60	115	20
Saltines	2 crackers	26	80	8
Noodles - enriched - cooked without salt	½ cup	100	T*	35
Spaghetti - enriched - cooked (firm) without salt	½ cup	80	T*	43
White bread - enriched	1 slice	64	123	27
Whole wheat bread	1 slice	61	129	33
Soups - Canned, Condensed, Made with Water				
Chicken Noodle	1 cup	75	1107	55

Tomato	1 cup	160	932	450
Vegetable Beef	1 cup	79	957	173
Fats				
Salt pork - raw	1 oz.	212	404	19
Corn Oil	1 Tbsp.	120	0	0
Soybean Oil	1 Tbsp.	120	0	0
Vegetable Shortening	1 Tbsp.	106	0	0
Fruits and juices				
Apple - raw, whole	1 medium	81	1	159
Avocado, raw, peeled	1 medium	306	21	1097
Banana, raw	1 medium	105	1	451
Cantaloupe, raw	1 cup	57	14	494
Nectarines, raw	1 medium	67	0	288
Orange, whole	1 medium	65	1	250
Peaches, raw	1 medium	37	0	171
Pears, raw	1 medium	98	1	208
Pineapple, canned, juice pack	½ cup	75	2	152
Raisins - dried, seedless	1 Tbsp.	29	3	76
Strawberries, raw, whole	1 cup	45	2	247
Watermelon balls/cubes	1 cup	50	3	186
Apple juice - canned	½ cup	58	3	148
Orange juice - frozen, unsweetened	½ cup	56	1	237
Tomato juice - canned	½ cup	22	439	267
Vegetables				
Green beans - canned	½ cup	13	170	74
Broccoli - cooked	½ cup	23	8	127
Cabbage	½ cup	16	14	154
Carrots - canned	½ cup	35	176	131
Cauliflower - cooked	½ cup	15	4	200
Collard greens - cooked	½ cup	31	42	214
Sweet potatoes - baked	1 small	188	12	397
White potatoes - baked	1 medium	220	16	844
Celery - raw	½ cup	6	35	114
Tomato - raw	1 medium	24	10	254
Peas, canned	⅓ cup	59	186	147
Spinach - canned	½ cup	25	29	370
Corn - canned	½ cup	83	286	192
Milk				
Cow - fluid - buttermilk from skim milk	1 cup	99	257	371
Cow - skim	1 cup	86	126	406
Cow - whole (3/5% fat)	1 cup	150	122	351
Meat				
Beef - chuck - ground, cooked	3 ½ oz.	159	56	359
Lamb - loin chop - lean marbled, cooked	3 oz.	255	38	175
Luncheon meat - beef bologna	1 slice	72	226	36

Pork				
Bacon - cured - broiled or fried	3 slices	109	303	92
Ham - cured, but lean, cooked	½ oz.	286	1072	258
Pork - loin chop - lean, cooked	3 ½ oz.	346	66	351
Sausage link - cooked	1 link	48	168	47
Poultry, eggs				
Chicken - roasted light meat without skin, chopped	3 oz.	190	86	243
Turkey - light meat, roasted	3 ½ oz.	157	64	305
Eggs - chicken - whole fresh	1 large	79	69	65
Egg substitute - Fleishman's Egg Beaters	¼ cup	96	120	128
Fish				
Bass, baked (1 serving)	4 oz.	287	68	256
Salmon - pink - canned	3 oz.	118	471	277
Shrimp - cooked	3 oz.	84	190	154
Tuna - canned, chunk-style in oil	3 oz.	245	679	256
Cheese				
American, processed	1 oz.	106	406	46
Cheddar	1 oz.	114	176	28
Cottage, creamed	1 cup	217	850	177
Cream	1 oz. (2 T)	99	84	34
Mozzarella	1 oz.	80	106	19
Swiss	1 oz.	107	74	31

*Trace - less than 1 mg.

Source: Pennington, Jean, Douglass. Judith S. Bowes and Church's Food Values for Portions Commonly Used, 18th edition, J.B. Lippincot, Williams & Willkins, 2004.

LACTOSE CONTAINING FOODS*

Milk, yogurt, cheese, ice cream, ice milk, sherbet, and even butter contain lactose--amounts vary, with milk, yogurt, and cheese having the highest levels

Milk and milk products are often added to processed foods—foods that have been altered to prolong their shelf life. People with lactose intolerance should be aware of the many food products that may contain even small amounts of lactose, such as

- bread and other baked goods
- waffles, pancakes, biscuits, cookies, and mixes to make them
- processed breakfast foods such as doughnuts, frozen waffles and pancakes, toaster pastries, and sweet rolls
- processed breakfast cereals
- instant potatoes, soups, and breakfast drinks
- potato chips, corn chips, and other processed snacks
- processed meats, such as bacon, sausage, hot dogs, and lunch meats
- margarine
- salad dressings
- liquid and powdered milk-based meal replacements
- protein powders and bars
- candies
- non-dairy liquid and powdered coffee creamers
- non-dairy whipped toppings

Lactose is also used in some prescription medicines, including birth control pills, and over-the-counter medicines like products to treat stomach acid and gas. These medicines most often cause symptoms in people with severe lactose intolerance.

*National Digestive Diseases Clearinghouse

COMMON ABBREVIATIONS

a	before	GI	gastrointestinal
ABW	actual body weight	gm	gram
ac	before meals	GSW	Gun Shot Wound
ad lib, AD	as desired		
AHA	American Heart Association	HB, Hb or	hemoglobin
as tol	as tolerated	Hgb	
ASHD	arteriosclerotic heart disease	HBP	high blood pressure
BCAA	branched chain amino acids	HBV	high biological value
BEE	basal energy expenditure	Hct	hematocrit
BMR	basal metabolic rate	HDL	high density lipoprotein
BP	blood pressure	Ht	height
BSA	body surface area	HTN	hypertension
BT	bedtime	Hx	history
BUN	blood urea nitrogen	I & O	intake and output
c̄	with		
ca	approximately	IM	intramuscular
Ca	calcium	in	inches
Kcal	calorie	IV	intravenous
CHD	coronary heart disease	K	potassium
CHF	congestive heart failure	Kcal (Kcal)	kilocalories
CHO	carbohydrate	kg	kilogram
Chol	cholesterol	L or l	liter
Cl	chloride	lb	pound
COPD	chronic obstructive pulmonary	LBV	low biological value
	disease	LDL	low density lipoprotein
CRF	chronic renal failure	LDN	licensed dietitian/nutritionist
CVA	cardiovascular accident		
DB or db	diabetic		
DBW	desirable body weight	mcg	microgram
DM	diabetes mellitus	mEq	milliequivalent
dp	diastolic pressure	mg	milligram
Dx	diagnosis	Mg	magnesium
ea	each	MI	myocardial infarction
ECG or EKG	electrocardiogram	mL	milliliter
EEG	electroencephalogram	MOsm	milliosmole
EFA	essential fatty acid	Na	sodium
ESRD	end stage renal disease	NaCl	salt, sodium chloride
FBS	fasting blood sugar	NPN	nonprotein nitrogen
FDA	Food and Drug Administration	NPO	nothing by mouth
Fe	iron	NR	not remarkable
FF	fat free		
GB	gallbladder		

oz	ounce	RDA	recommended dietary allowance
P	phosphorus		reduction
pc	after eating/meals	red	resting energy expenditure
		REE	resting metabolic rate
		RMR	

PD	peritoneal dialysis	$\bar{s}$	without
per diem	per day	SA	serum albumin
PKU	phenylketonuria	SDA	specific dynamic action
PN	parental nutrition	SF	salt free
po	postoperative or by mouth	SBP	systolic blood pressure
PPN	peripheral parenteral nutrition	stat	at once
		TAH	total abdominal hysterectomy
PRN	as requested/needed	TB	tuberculosis
pro	protein	Tbsp, T	tablespoon
Pt	patient	TID or tid	three times a day
pt	pint	TLC	total lymphocyte count
PVD	peripheral vascular disease	TP	total protein
PZI	protamine zinc insulin	tsp, t	teaspoon
QID	four times daily	UBW	usual body weight
qt	quart	URI	upper respiratory infection
RBC	red blood count	UTI	urinary tract infection
RD	registered dietitian	WBC	white blood count
		wt, W	weight
		Zn	zinc

Also note the Joint Commission list of "Do Not Use" Abbreviations. This list is updated annually.

Prefixes		Suffixes	
chol-	gallbladder related	-ectomy	removal of
gastr-	stomach related	-itis	inflammation of
hyper-	elevated, above normal	-oma	tumor related
hypo-	reduced, below normal	-scopy	examination of

Common Measurements

Table of Weights and Measures

Weight	Length
1 ounce = 38 grams 1 pound = 453.6 grams 1 microgram = 0.001 milligram 1 milligram = 0.001 gram 1 gram = 0.035 ounces or 0.001 kilogram 1 kilogram = 2.2 pounds or 1000 grams	1 inch = 2.54 centimeters 1 foot = 12 inches 1 yard = 3 feet 1 millimeter = 0.4 inches 1 meter = 1.1 yards

Volume

1 teaspoon = 5 mL
1 tablespoon = 15 mL or 3 teaspoons
1 fluid ounce = 30 mL
1 cup = 8 fluid ounces or 240 mL or 16 tablespoons
2 cups = 1 pint
3 pints = 1 quart
4 quarts = 1 gallon
2 gallons = 1 peck
4 pecks = 1 bushel
1 liter = 1.06 quarts

Approximate Conversion to Metric Measures

Given:	Multiply by:	To determine:
ounces (oz)	28.0	grams (gm)
pounds (lb)	0.45	kilograms (kg)
teaspoons (t; tsp)	5.0	milliliters (mL)
tablespoons (T; Tbsp)	15.0	milliliters (mL)
fluid ounces (oz)	30.0	milliliters (mL)
cups (c)	0.24	liters (L)
pints (pt)	0.47	liters (L)
quarts (qt)	0.95	liters (L)
gallons (gal)	3.8	liters (L)

Kilocalorie Values Of Energy Containing Nutrients

1 gm protein	=	4 kilocalories
1 gm carbohydrate	=	4 kilocalories
1 gm fat	=	9 kilocalories
1 gm alcohol	=	7 kilocalories

LITERATURE CITED

Nutrition Assessment

1. Frankenfield D, Roth-Yousey L, Compher C. Comparison of predictive equations for resting metabolic rate in healthy nonobese and obese adults: a systematic review. *J Am Diet Assoc.* 2005;105(5):775-89.
2. Walker R, Heubberger R. Predictive Equations for Energy Needs for the Critically Ill. *Respr Care.* 2009; 54, 509-521.
3. Dietary Reference Intakes for Energy, Carbohydrate, Fiber, Fat, Fatty Acids, Cholesterol, Protein, and Amino Acids (Macronutrients). Food and Nutrition Board (FNB) of the Institute of Medicine. National Academies Press. 2011. Accessed January 21, 2015
4. Mifflin MD, St Jeor ST, Hill LA, Scott BJ, Daugherty SA, Koh YO. A new predictive equation for resting energy expenditure in healthy individuals. *Am J Clin Nutr.* 1990;51(2):241-247.
5. Boullata J, Williams J, Cottrell F, Hudson L, Compher C. Accurate determination of energy needs in hospitalized patients. *J Am Diet Assoc.* 2007;107(3):393-401.
6. Amirkalali B, Hosseini S, Heshmat R, Larijani B. Comparison of Harris Benedict and Mifflin-ST Jeor equations with indirect calorimetry in evaluating resting energy expenditure. *Indian J Med Sci.* 2008;62(7):283-90.
7. Japur CC, Penaforte FR, Chiarello PG, Monteiro JP, Vieira MN, Basile-Filho A. Harris-Benedict equation for critically ill patients: Are there differences with indirect calorimetry? *J Crit Care.* 2009 Feb 11.
8. National Heart Lung and Blood Institute. Clinical Guidelines on the Identification, Evaluation, and Treatment of Overweight and Obesity in Adults: The Evidence Report. Accessed January 21, 2015.
9. Winter J, MacInnis R, Wattanapenpaiboon N, Nowson C. BMI and all-cause mortality in older adults: a meta-analysis. *The American Journal of Clinical Nutrition*; 2014: ajcn-068122.
10. Chau D, Cho LM, Jani P, St Jeor ST. Individualizing recommendations for weight management in the elderly. *Curr Opin Clin Nutr Metab Care.* 2008 ;11(1):27-31.
11. Chumlea WC, Gui SS, Steinbaugh ML. Prediction of stature from knee height for black and white adults and children with application to mobility-impaired or handicapped persons. *J Am Diet Assoc.* 1994;94:1385-1388.
12. Chumlea WC, Guo SS, Wholihan K, Cockram D, Kuczmarski RJ, Johnson CL. Stature prediction equations for elderly non-Hispanic white, non-Hispanic black, and Mexican-American persons developed from NHANES III data. *J Am Diet Assoc.* 1998 Feb;98(2):137-42.
13. Van Lier AM, Roy MA, Payette H. Knee height to predict stature in North American Caucasian frail free-living elderly receiving community services. *J Nutr Health Aging.* 2007;11:372-9.

14. Pini R, Tonon E, Cavallini MC, Bencini F, Di Bari M, Masotti G, Marchionni N. Accuracy of equations for predicting stature from knee height, and assessment of statural loss in an older Italian population. *J Gerontol A Biol Sci Med Sci.* 2001;56(1):B3-7.

15. Shahar S, Pooy NS. Predictive equations for estimation of stature in Malaysian elderly people. *Asia Pac J Clin Nutr.* 2003;12(1):80-4.

16. Ozer BK, Gültekin T, Sağir M. Estimation of stature in Turkish adults using knee height. *Anthropol Anz.* 2007;65(2):213-22.

17. Zhang H, Hsu-Hage BH, Wahlqvist ML. The use of knee height to estimate maximum stature in elderly Chinese. *J Nutr Health Aging.* 1998;2(2):84-7.

18. Hickson M, Frost G. A comparison of three methods for estimating height in the acutely ill elderly population. *J Hum Nutr Diet.* 2003;16(1):13-20.

19. Greenwood J, Narus S, Leiser J, Egger M. Measuring body index according to protocol: how are height and weight obtained. J Health Qual. 2011; 33:28-36.

20. Cockram DB, Baumgartner RN. Evaluation of accuracy and reliability of calipers for measuring recumbent knee height in elderly people. *Am J Clin Nutr.* 1990;52(2):397-400.

21. Nelms M, Sucher K, Long S. Nutrition Therapy and Pathophysiology. 2007. Belmont California. Thompson Wadsworth.

22. Hume P, Marfell-Jones M. The importance of accurate site location for skinfold measurement. *J Sports Sci.* 2008;26(12):1333-40.

23. Orphanidou C, McCargar L, Birmingham CL, Mathieson J, Goldner E. Accuracy of subcutaneous fat measurement: comparison of skinfold calipers, ultrasound, and computed tomography. *J Am Diet Assoc.* 1994;94(8):855-8.

24. Klein S, Kinney J, Jeejeebhoy K, Alpers D, Hellerstein M, Murray M, Twomey P. Nutrition support in clinical practice: review of published data and recommendations for future research directions. Summary of a conference sponsored by the National Institutes of Health, American Society for Parenteral and Enteral Nutrition, and American Society for Clinical Nutrition. *Am J Clin Nutr.* 1997;66(3):683-706.

25. Chumlea WC, Roche AF, Mukherjee D. Nutritional assessment of the elderly through anthropometry. 1987. Columbus, OH. Ross Laboratories.

26. Chumlea WC, Roche AF. Assessment of the nutritional status of healthy and handicapped adults. In: Lohman TG, Roche AF, Martorell R (eds). Anthropometric standardization reference manual. 1988. Champaign, IL. Human Kinetics Books.

27. Grundy SM, Cleeman JI, Daniels SR, et al. Diagnosis and management of the metabolic syndrome: an American Heart Association/National Heart, Lung, and Blood Instititute Scientific Statement. *Circulation.* 2005; 112: 2735-52.

28. Rosenzweig J, Ferrannini E, Grundy S, et al. Primary prevention of cardiovascular disease and type 2 diabetes in patients at metabolic risk: an endocrine society clinical practice guideline. *J Clin Endocrinol Metab.* 2008; 93: 3671-89.

29. Keller HH, Gibbs-Ward A, Randall-Simpson J, Bocock MA, Dimou E. Meal rounds: an essential aspect of quality nutrition services in long-term care. *J Am Med Dir Assoc.* 2006;7(1):40-45.

30. Simmons SF, Babineau S, Garcia E, Schnelle JF. Quality assessment in nursing homes by systematic direct observation: feeding assistance. *J Gerontol A Biol Sci Med Sci.* 2002;57(10):M665-671.

31. Schnelle JF, Osterweil D, Simmons SF. Improving the quality of nursing home care and medical-record accuracy with direct observational technologies. *Gerontologist.* 2005;45(5):576-82.

Regular and Mechanically Altered Diets

1. U.S. Department of Health and Human Services and U.S. Department of Agriculture. Dietary Guidelines for Americans, 2015. 8th Edition, Washington, DC: U.S. Government Printing Office, June 2015.
2. U.S. Department of Agriculture. MyPlate. Accessed January 21, 2015.
3. Johnson LE, Dooley PA, Gleick JB. Oral nutritional supplement use in elderly nursing home patients. *J Am Geriatr Soc.* 1993;41(9):947-952.
4. Arnaud-Battandier F, Malvy D, Jeandel C, Schmitt C, Aussage P, Beaufrère B, Cynober L. Use of oral supplements in malnourished elderly patients living in the community: a pharmaco-economic study. *Clin Nutr.* 2004;23(5):1096-1103.
5. Manders M, de Groot CP, Blauw YH, Dhonukshe-Rutten RA, van Hoeckel-Prüst L, Bindels JG, Siebelink E, van Staveren WA. Effect of a nutrient-enriched drink on dietary intake and nutritional status in institutionalised elderly. *Eur J Clin Nutr.* 2009 May 20.
6. Ross F. An audit of nutritional supplement distribution and consumption on a care of the elderly ward. *J Hum Nutr Diet.* 1999;12:445-452.
7. Wilson M-MG, Purushothaman R, Morley JE. Effect of liquid dietary supplements on energy intake in the elderly. *Am J Clin Nutr.* 2002;75:944-947.
8. Whiteman E, Ward K, Simmons SF, Sarkisian CA, Moore AA. Testing the effect of specific orders to provide oral liquid nutritional supplements to nursing home residents: a quality improvement project. *J Nutr Health Aging.* 2008;12(9):622-625.
9. Zak M, Swine C, Grodzicki T. Combined effects of functionally-oriented exercise regimens and nutritional supplementation on both the institutionalised and free-living frail elderly (double-blind, randomised clinical trial). *BMC Public Health.* 2009;9:39.
10. Castellanos VH, Marra MV, Johnson P. Enhancement of select foods at breakfast and lunch increases energy intakes of nursing home residents with low meal intakes. *J Am Diet Assoc.* 2009;109(3):445-451.
11. Silver HJ, Dietrich MS, Castellanos VH. Increased energy density of the home-delivered lunch meal improves 24-hour nutrient intakes in older adults. *J Am Diet Assoc.* 2008;108(12):2084-9.
12. Bernstein MA, Tucker KL, Ryan ND, O'Neill EF, Clements KM, Nelson ME, Evans WJ, Fiatarone Singh MA. Higher dietary variety is associated with better nutritional status in frail elderly people. *J Am Diet Assoc.* 2002;102(8):1096-1104.
13. Bermejo LM, Aparicio A, Andrés P, López-Sobaler AM, Ortega RM. The influence of fruit and vegetable intake on the nutritional status and plasma homocysteine levels of institutionalised elderly people. *Public Health Nutr.* 2007;10(3):266-272.
14. Simmons SF, Keeler E, Zhuo X, Hickey KA, Sato HW, Schnelle JF. Prevention of unintentional weight loss in nursing home residents: a controlled trial of feeding assistance. *J Am Geriatr Soc.* 2008;56(8):1466-1473.

15. Simmons SF, Schnelle JF. Individualized feeding assistance care for nursing home residents: staffing requirements to implement two interventions. *J Gerontol A Biol Sci Med Sci.* 2004;59(9):M966-973.

16. Simmons SF, Osterweil D, Schnelle JF. Improving food intake in nursing home residents with feeding assistance: a staffing analysis. *J Gerontol A Biol Sci Med Sci.* 2001;56(12):M790-94.

17. Gustashaw K. Position of the Academy of Nutrition and Dietetics: Individualized nutrition approaches for adults in health care communities. 2010; 110(10): 1554-1563.

18. Bartali B, Salvini S, Turrini A, Lauretani F, Russo CR, Corsi AM, Bandinelli S, D'Amicis A, Palli D, Guralnik JM, Ferrucci L. Age and disability affect dietary intake. *J Nutr.* 2003;133(9):2868-2873.

19. Syme S. Independence through finger food. Contemp Nursing 2005;4:80-81.

20. Jean LA. "Finger food menu" restores independence in dining. *Health Care Food Nutr Focus* 1997;14:4-6.

21. Dahl WJ, Whiting SJ, Tyler RT. Protein content of puréed diets: implications for planning. *Can J Diet Pract Res.* 2007;68(2):99-102.

22. Adolphe JL, Whiting SL, Dahl WJ. Vitamin fortification of puréed foods for long-term care residents. *Can J Diet Pract Res.* 2009;70(3):143-50.

23. The National Dyshagia Diet. https://www.dysphagia-diet.com/t-resources.aspx Accessed January 21, 2015.

Reduced Sodium Diet

1. Paterna S, Parrinello G, Cannizzaro S, Fasullo S, Torres D, Sarullo FM, Di Pasquale P. Medium term effects of different dosage of diuretic, sodium, and fluid administration on neurohormonal and clinical outcome in patients with recently compensated heart failure. *Am J Cardiol.* 2009;103(1):93-102.

2. Kollipara UK, Jaffer O, Amin A, Toto KH, Nelson LL, Schneider R, Markham D, Drazner MH. Relation of lack of knowledge about dietary sodium to hospital readmission in patients with heart failure. *Am J Cardiol.* 2008;102(9):1212-5.

3. Arcand JA, Brazel S, Joliffe C, Choleva M, Berkoff F, Allard JP, Newton GE. Education by a dietitian in patients with heart failure results in improved adherence with a sodium-restricted diet: a randomized trial. *Am Heart J.* 2005;150(4):716.

4. Alvelos M, Ferreira A, Bettencourt P, Serrão P, Pestana M, Cerqueira-Gomes M, Soares-Da-Silva P. The effect of dietary sodium restriction on neurohumoral activity and renal dopaminergic response in patients with heart failure. *Eur J Heart Fail.* 2004;6(5):593-9.

5. Academy of Nutrition and Dietetics Evidence Analysis Library. Hypertension. Academy of Nutrition and Dietetics, Accessed 01 August 2015, http://www.andeal.org/topic.cfm?menu=5285&pcat=3260&cat=5413.

6. Paterna S, Gaspare P, Fasullo S, Sarullo FM, Di Pasquale P. Normal-sodium diet compared with low-sodium diet in compensated congestive heart failure: is sodium an old enemy or a new friend? *Clin Sci (Lond).* 2008;114(3):221-30.

7. Beich KR, Yancy C. The heart failure and sodium restriction controversy: challenging conventional practice. *Nutr Clin Pract.* 2008;23(5):477-486.

8. Tuttle KR, Sunwold D, Kramer H. Can comprehensive lifestyle change alter the course of chronic kidney disease? *Semin Nephrol.* 2009;29(5):512-523.

9. Krikken JA, Laverman GD, Navis G. Benefits of dietary sodium restriction in the management of chronic kidney disease. *Curr Opin Nephrol Hypertens.* 2009 Jun 26.

10. Ritz E, Koleganova N, Piecha G. Role of sodium intake in the progression of chronic kidney disease. *J Ren Nutr.* 2009;19(1):61-62.

11. Ritz E, Mehls O. Salt restriction in kidney disease--a missed therapeutic opportunity? Pediatr Nephrol. 2009;24(1):9-17.

12. Kayikcioglu M, Tumuklu M, Ozkahya M, Ozdogan O, Asci G, Duman S, Toz H, Can LH, Basci A, Ok E. The benefit of salt restriction in the treatment of end-stage renal disease by haemodialysis. *Nephrol Dial Transplant.* 2009;24(3):956-962.

13. Sanders PW. Assessment and treatment of hypertension in dialysis: the case for salt restriction. *Semin Dial.* 2007;20(5):408-411.

14. Lee L, Grap MJ. Care and management of the patient with ascites. *Medsurg Nurs.* 2008;17(6):376-381; quiz 382.

15. Sargent S. The management and nursing care of cirrhotic ascites. *Br J Nurs.* 2006;15(4):212-219.

16. Ginès P, Cárdenas A. The management of ascites and hyponatremia in cirrhosis. *Semin Liver Dis.* 2008;28(1):43-58.

17. Møller S, Henriksen JH, Bendtsen F. Pathogenetic background for treatment of ascites and hepatorenal syndrome. *Hepatol Int.* 2008;2(4):416-428.

18. Møller S, Henriksen JH, Bendtsen F. Ascites: Pathogenesis and therapeutic principles. *Scand J Gastroenterol.* 2009 May 28:1-10.

19. Kashani A, Landaverde C, Medici V, Rossaro L. Fluid retention in cirrhosis: pathophysiology and management. *QJM.* 2008;101(2):71-85. Epub 2008 Jan 9.

20. Burns ER, Neubort S. Sodium content of koshered meat. *JAMA.* 1984;252:2960.

21. Glick SM. Salt content of kosher meat. *JAMA.* 1985; 254:504.

22. Kisch B. Salt poor diets and Jewish dietary laws. *JAMA.* 1953;153:1472.

23. Academy of Nutrition and Dietetics Evidence Analysis Library. *Hypertension.* Academy of Nutrition and Dietetics, Accessed 12 January 2015, http://www.andeal.org/topic.cfm?menu=5285&cat=3261.

24. Levitan EB, Wolk A, Mittleman MA. Consistency with the DASH diet and incidence of heart failure. *Arch Intern Med.* 2009;169(9):851-857.

25. Kotchen TA. Does the DASH diet improve clinical outcomes in hypertensive patients? *Am J Hypertens.* 2009 Apr;22(4):350.

26. Jacobs DR Jr, Gross MD, Steffen L, Steffes MW, Yu X, Svetkey LP, Appel LJ, Vollmer WM, Bray GA, Moore T, Conlin PR, Sacks F. The effects of dietary patterns on urinary albumin excretion: results of the Dietary Approaches to Stop Hypertension (DASH) Trial. *Am J Kidney Dis.* 2009;53(4):638-46.

27. Jehn ML, Brotman DJ, Appel LJ. Racial differences in diurnal blood pressure and heart rate patterns: results from the Dietary Approaches to Stop Hypertension (DASH) trial. *Arch Intern Med.* 2008;168(9):996-1002.

28. Lin PH, Appel LJ, Funk K, Craddick S, Chen C, Elmer P, McBurnie MA, Champagne C. The PREMIER intervention helps participants follow the Dietary Approaches to Stop

Hypertension dietary pattern and the current Dietary Reference Intakes recommendations. *J Am Diet Assoc.* 2007;107(9):1541-1551.

29. Folsom AR, Parker ED, Harnack LJ. Degree of concordance with DASH diet guidelines and incidence of hypertension and fatal cardiovascular disease. *Am J Hypertens.* 2007;20(3):225-32.

30. Miller ER 3rd, Erlinger TP, Appel LJ. The effects of macronutrients on blood pressure and lipids: an overview of the DASH and OmniHeart trials. *Curr Atheroscler Rep.* 2006;8(6):460-465.

31. Champagne CM. Dietary interventions on blood pressure: the Dietary Approaches to Stop Hypertension (DASH) trials. *Nutr Rev.* 2006;64(2 Pt 2):S53-56.

32. Most MM. Estimated phytochemical content of the dietary approaches to stop hypertension (DASH) diet is higher than in the Control Study Diet. *J Am Diet Assoc.* 2004;104(11):1725-1727.

33. Bray GA, Vollmer WM, Sacks FM, Obarzanek E, Svetkey LP, Appel LJ; DASH Collaborative Research Group. A further subgroup analysis of the effects of the DASH diet and three dietary sodium levels on blood pressure: results of the DASH-Sodium Trial. *Am J Cardiol.* 2004;94(2):222-227.

34. He FJ, MacGregor GA. Potassium: more beneficial effects. *Climacteric.* 2003;6 Suppl 3:36-48.

35. Most MM, Craddick S, Crawford S, Redican S, Rhodes D, Rukenbrod F, Laws R; Dash-Sodium Collaborative Research Group. Dietary quality assurance processes of the DASH-Sodium controlled diet study. *J Am Diet Assoc.* 2003;103(10):1339-1346.

36. Lin PH, Aickin M, Champagne C, Craddick S, Sacks FM, McCarron P, Most-Windhauser MM, Rukenbrod F, Haworth L; Dash-Sodium Collaborative Research Group. Food group sources of nutrients in the dietary patterns of the DASH-Sodium trial. *J Am Diet Assoc.* 2003;103(4):488-496.

37. Frank GC. The DASH diet. A practical tool for hypertension management in the elderly. *Adv Nurse Pract.* 2001;9(7):57-60.

38. Vollmer WM, Sacks FM, Svetkey LP. New insights into the effects on blood pressure of diets low in salt and high in fruits and vegetables and low-fat dairy products. *Curr Control Trials Cardiovasc Med.* 2001;2(2):71-74.

39. Moore TJ, Conlin PR, Ard J, Svetkey LP. DASH (Dietary Approaches to Stop Hypertension) diet is effective treatment for stage 1 isolated systolic hypertension. *Hypertension.* 2001;38(2):155-158.

40. Sacks FM, Svetkey LP, Vollmer WM, Appel LJ, Bray GA, Harsha D, Obarzanek E, Conlin PR, Miller ER 3rd, Simons-Morton DG, Karanja N, Lin PH; DASH-Sodium Collaborative Research Group. Effects on blood pressure of reduced dietary sodium and the Dietary Approaches to Stop Hypertension (DASH) diet. DASH-Sodium Collaborative Research Group. *N Engl J Med.* 2001;344(1):3-10.

41. Conlin PR, Chow D, Miller ER 3rd, Svetkey LP, Lin PH, Harsha DW, Moore TJ, Sacks FM, Appel LJ. The effect of dietary patterns on blood pressure control in hypertensive patients: results from the Dietary Approaches to Stop Hypertension (DASH) trial. *Am J Hypertens.* 2000;13(9):949-955.

42. Appel LJ, Moore TJ, Obarzanek E, Vollmer WM, Svetkey LP, Sacks FM, Bray GA, Vogt TM, Cutler JA, Windhauser MM, Lin PH, Karanja N. A clinical trial of the effects

of dietary patterns on blood pressure. DASH Collaborative Research Group. *N Engl J Med.* 1997;336(16):1117-1124.

43. National Heart, Lung, and Blood Institute. Your Guide to Lowering Your Blood Pressure With DASH — A Week With the DASH Eating Plan. Retrieved 05, August 2015: http://www.nhlbi.nih.gov/health/resources/heart/hbp-dash-week-dash-html.

Cardiovascular Management

1. Vannice G, Rasmussen H, *Position of the Academy of Nutrition and Dietetics: dietary fatty acids for healthy adults.* Journal of the Academy of Nutrition and Dietetics. 2014: 114 (1): 136-153.

2. National Cholesterol Education Program (NCEP) Expert Panel on Detection, Evaluation, and Treatment of High Blood Cholesterol in Adults (Adult Treatment Panel III). *Third report of the National Cholesterol Education Program (NCEP) Expert Panel on Detection, Evaluation, and Treatment of High Blood Cholesterol in Adults (Adult Treatment Panel III) final report.* Circulation. 2002; 106 (25):3143-3421.

3. Appel LJ, et al. Diet and lifestyle recommendations revision 2006: *A scientific statement from the American Heart Association nutrition committee.* Circulation. 2006; 114 (1):82-96.

Diabetes

1. Tariq SH, Karcic E, Thomas DR, Thomson K, Philpot C, Chapel DL, Morley JE. The use of a no-concentrated-sweets diet in the management of type 2 diabetes in nursing homes. *J Am Diet Assoc.* 2001;101(12):1463-1466.

2. Diabetes Nutrition Recommendations for Health Care Institutions (translation). *Diabetes Care* 1999;22:S46-S48.

3. Daly A, et al. *Exchange lists for diabetes.* The American Diabetes Association. 2008.

Gastrointestinal Diets

1. National Institute of Diabetes, Digestive, and Kidney Diseases (NIDDK). Diarrhea. Retrieved 05 August 2015. http://www.niddk.nih.gov/health-information/health-topics/digestive-diseases/diarrhea/Pages/facts.aspx

2. Lomer MC, Parkes GC, Sanderson JD. Review article: lactose intolerance in clinical practice--myths and realities. *Aliment Pharmacol Ther.* 2008;27(2):93-103.

3. Ventura E, Davis J, Byrd-Williams C, Alexander K, McClain A, Lane CJ, Spruijt-Metz D, Weigensberg M, Goran M. Reduction in risk factors for type 2 diabetes mellitus in response to a low-sugar, high-fiber dietary intervention in overweight Latino adolescents. *Arch Pediatr Adolesc Med.* 2009;163(4):320-327.

4. Rovner AJ, Nansel TR, Gellar L. The effect of a low-glycemic diet vs a standard diet on blood glucose levels and macronutrient intake in children with type 1 diabetes. *J Am Diet Assoc.* 2009;109(2):303-307.

5. Livesey G, Tagami H. Interventions to lower the glycemic response to carbohydrate foods with a low-viscosity fiber (resistant maltodextrin): meta-analysis of randomized controlled trials. *Am J Clin Nutr.* 2009;89(1):114-125.

6. Jenkins AL, Jenkins DJ, Wolever TM, Rogovik AL, Jovanovski E, Bozikov V, Rahelić D, Vuksan V. Comparable postprandial glucose reductions with viscous fiber blend enriched biscuits in healthy subjects and patients with diabetes mellitus: acute randomized controlled clinical trial. *Croat Med J.* 2008;49(6):772-782.

7. Alminger M, Eklund-Jonsson C. Whole-grain cereal products based on a high-fibre barley or oat genotype lower post-prandial glucose and insulin responses in healthy humans. *Eur J Nutr.* 2008;47(6):294-300.

8. Theuwissen E, Mensink RP. Water-soluble dietary fibers and cardiovascular disease. *Physiol Behav.* 2008;94(2):285-292.

9. Sadiq Butt M, Tahir-Nadeem M, Khan MK, Shabir R, Butt MS. Oat: unique among the cereals. *Eur J Nutr.* 2008;47(2):68-79.

10. Wu K, Bowman R, Welch AA, Luben RN, Wareham N, Khaw KT, Bingham SA. Apolipoprotein E polymorphisms, dietary fat and fibre, and serum lipids: the EPIC Norfolk study. *Eur Heart J.* 2007;28(23):2930-2936.

11. Finley JW, Burrell JB, Reeves PG. Pinto bean consumption changes SCFA profiles in fecal fermentations, bacterial populations of the lower bowel, and lipid profiles in blood of humans. *J. Nutr.* 2007;137(11):2391-2398.

12. Aleixandre A, Miguel M. Dietary fiber in the prevention and treatment of metabolic syndrome: a review. *Crit Rev Food Sci Nutr.* 2008;48(10):905-912.

13. Galisteo M, Duarte J, Zarzuelo A. Effects of dietary fibers on disturbances clustered in the metabolic syndrome. *J Nutr Biochem.* 2008;19(2):71-84.

14. Anderson JW, Baird P, Davis RH Jr, Ferreri S, Knudtson M, Koraym A, Waters V, Williams CL. Health benefits of dietary fiber. *Nutr Rev.* 2009;67(4):188-205.

15. Bortolotti M, Levorato M, Lugli A, Mazzero G. Effect of a balanced mixture of dietary fibers on gastric emptying, intestinal transit and body weight. *Ann Nutr Metab.* 2008;52(3):221-226.

16. Slavin J. *Position of the American Dietetic Association: health implications of dietary fiber.* 2008:108(10); 1716-1731.

17. Floch MH, White JA. Management of diverticular disease is changing. *World Journal of Gastroenterology.* 2006;12(20):3225-3228.

18. Janes SEJ, Meagher A, Frizelle FA. Management of diverticulitis. *BMJ Medical Publication of the Year.* 2006;332:271-275.

19. Aldoori W, Ryan-Harshman M. Preventing diverticular disease: Review of recent evidence on high-fibre diets. *Canadian Family Physician.* 2002;48:1632-1637.

20. Grabitske HA, Slavin JL. Low-Digestible Carbohydrates in Practice. *J Am Diet Assoc.* 2008;108:1677-1681.

21. Strate L, Liu Y, Syngal S, Aldoori W, Giovannucci E. Nut, Corn, and Popcorn Consumption and the Incidence of Diverticular Disease. *JAMA.* 2008;300(8):907-914.

22. Marcason W. What is the latest research regarding the avoidance of nuts, seeds, corn, and popcorn in diverticular disease? *J Am Diet Assoc.* 2008;108(11):1956.

23. Weisberger L, Jamieson B. Clinical inquiries: How can you help prevent a recurrence of diverticulitis? *J Fam Pract.* 2009;58(7):381-382.

24. Radigan, A. E. Post-Gastrectomy: Managing the nutrition fall-out. *Practical Gastroenterology.* 2004; 18: 63-75.
25. Fujioka, K. Follow-up of nutritional and metabolic problems after Bariatric surgery. *Diabetes Care.* 2005;28(2):481-484.
26. Beyan C. Post-gastrectomy Anemia: evaluation of 72 cases with post-gastrectomy anemia. *Hematology.* Feb. 2007;12(1):81-84.
27. Pawson R, Mehta A. Review article: the diagnosis and treatment of haematinic deficiency in gastrointestinal disease. *Alimentary Pharmocology and Therapeutics.* 1998;12:687-698.
28. Beyan C, Beyan E, Kaptan K, Ifran A, Uzar AI. Post-gastrectomy anemia: evaluation of 72 cases with post-gastrectomy anemia. *Hematology.* 2007;12(1):81-84.
29. Lim JS, Kim SB, Bang HY, Cheon GJ, Lee JI. High prevalence of osteoporosis in patients with gastric adenocarcinoma following gastrectomy. *World J Gastroenterol.* 2007;13(48):6492-6497.
30. Southerland JC, Valentine JF. Osteopenia and osteoporosis in gastrointestinal diseases: diagnosis and treatment. *Curr Gastroenterol Rep.* 2001;3(5):399-407.
31. Dickey W. Making oats safer for patients with coeliac disease. *Eur J Gastroenterol Hepatol.* 2008;20(6):494-495.
32. Ellis HJ, Ciclitira PJ. Should coeliac sufferers be allowed their oats? *Eur J Gastroenterol Hepatol.* 2008;20(6):492-493.
33. Sadiq Butt M, Tahir-Nadeem M, Khan MK, Shabir R, Butt MS. Oat: unique among the cereals. *Eur J Nutr.* 2008;47(2):68-79.
34. Guttormsen V, Løvik A, Bye A, Bratlie J, Mørkrid L, Lundin KE. No induction of anti-avenin IgA by oats in adult, diet-treated coeliac disease. *Scand J Gastroenterol.* 2008;43(2):161-165.
35. Rashid M, Butzner D, Burrows V, Zarkadas M, Case S, Molloy M, Warren R, Pulido O, Switzer C. Consumption of pure oats by individuals with celiac disease: a position statement by the Canadian Celiac Association. *Can J Gastroenterol.* 2007;21(10):649-651.

Renal Diets

1. National Kidney Foundation. K/DOKI guidelines for Nutrition in Chronic Renal Failure. Am J Kidney Dis. 2000; 35(6, Suppl 2): S1-S201.

HIV/AIDS

1. Oguntibeju OO, van den Heever WM, Van Schalkwyk FE. The interrelationship between nutrition and the immune system in HIV infection: a review. *Pak J Biol Sci.* 2007;10(24):4327-38.
2. Brown TT, Xu X, John M, Singh J, Kingsley LA, Palella FJ, Witt MD, Margolick JB, Dobs AS. Fat distribution and longitudinal anthropometric changes in HIV-infected men with and without clinical evidence of lipodystrophy and HIV-uninfected controls: a substudy of the Multicenter AIDS Cohort Study. *AIDS Res Ther.* 2009;13;6:8.
3. Shlay JC, Sharma S, Peng G, Gibert CL, Grunfeld C; Terry Beirn Community Programs for Clinical Research on AIDS (CPCRA); International Network for Strategic Initiatives

in Global HIV Trials (INSIGHT). The effect of individual antiretroviral drugs on body composition in HIV-infected persons initiating highly active antiretroviral therapy. *J Acquir Immune Defic Syndr.* 200951(3):298-304.

4. Wohl DA, Brown TT. Management of morphologic changes associated with antiretroviral use in HIV-infected patients. *J Acquir Immune Defic Syndr.* 2008;49 Suppl 2:S93-S100.

5. Aberg JA. Lipid management in patients who have HIV and are receiving HIV therapy. *Endocrinol Metab Clin North Am.* 2009;38(1):207-22.

6. Monsuez JJ, Charniot JC, Escaut L, Teicher E, Wyplosz B, Couzigou C, Vignat N, Vittecoq D. HIV-associated vascular diseases: structural and functional changes, clinical implications. *Int J Cardiol.* 2009;133(3):293-306.

7. Joy T, Keogh HM, Hadigan C, Lee H, Dolan SE, Fitch K, Liebau J, Lo J, Johnsen S, Hubbard J, Anderson EJ, Grinspoon S. Dietary fat intake and relationship to serum lipid levels in HIV-infected patients with metabolic abnormalities in the HAART era. *AIDS.* 2007;21(12):1591-600.

8. Jevtović DJ, Dragović G, Salemović D, Ranin J, Djurković-Djaković O. The metabolic syndrome, an epidemic among HIV-infected patients on HAART. *Biomed Pharmacother.* 2009;63(5):337-42.

9. Grunfeld C. Insulin resistance in HIV infection: drugs, host responses, or restoration to health? *Top HIV Med.* 2008;16(2):89-93.

10. Gkrania-Klotsas E, Klotsas AE. HIV and HIV treatment: effects on fats, glucose and lipids. *Br Med Bull.* 2007;84:49-68.

11. Dobbs MR, Berger JR. Stroke in HIV infection and AIDS. *Expert Rev Cardiovasc Ther.* 2009;7(10):1263-71.

12. Choi AI, Shlipak MG, Hunt PW, Martin JN, Deeks SG. HIV-infected persons continue to lose kidney function despite successful antiretroviral therapy. *AIDS.* 2009;23(16):2143-9.

13. Grund B, Peng G, Gibert CL, Hoy JF, Isaksson RL, Shlay JC, Martinez E, Reiss P, Visnegarwala F, Carr AD; INSIGHT SMART Body Composition Substudy Group. Continuous antiretroviral therapy decreases bone mineral density. *AIDS.* 2009;23(12):1519-29.

14. Gibert CL, Shlay JC, Sharma S, Bartsch G, Peng G, Grunfeld C; Terry Beirn Community Programs for Clinical Research on AIDS; International Network for Strategic Initiatives in Global HIV Trials. Racial differences in changes of metabolic parameters and body composition in antiretroviral therapy-naive persons initiating antiretroviral therapy. *J Acquir Immune Defic Syndr.* 2009;50(1):44-53.

Cancer

1. DeMille D, Deming P, Lupinacci P, Jacobs LA. The effect of the neutropenic diet in the outpatient setting: a pilot study. *Oncol Nurs Forum.* 2006;33(2):337-343.

2. Moody K, Finlay J, Mancuso C, Charlson M. Feasibility and safety of a pilot randomized trial of infection rate: neutropenic diet versus standard food safety guidelines. *J Pediatr Hematol Oncol.* 2006;28(3):126-133.

3. Moody K, Charlson ME, Finlay J. The neutropenic diet: what's the evidence? *J Pediatr Hematol Oncol.* 2002;24(9):717-721.
4. Restau J, Clark AP. The neutropenic diet: does the evidence support this intervention? *Clin Nurse Spec.* 2008;22(5):208-211.
5. Larson E, Nirenberg A. Evidence-based nursing practice to prevent infection in hospitalized neutropenic patients with cancer. *Oncol Nurs Forum.* 2004;31(4):717-725.

Enteral Nutrition

1. Boelens P, Nijveldt R, Houdijk A, Meijer S, van Leeuwen P. Glutamine Alimentation in Catabolic State. *Jour Nutr.* 2001; 131:2569S-2577S.
2. Vermeulen MA, van de Poll MC, Ligthart-Melis GC, Dejong CH, van den Tol MP, Boelens PG, van Leeuwen PA. Specific amino acids in the critically ill patient--exogenous glutamine/arginine: a common denominator? *Crit Care Med.* 2007 Sep;35(9 Suppl):S568-576.
3. Buchman, A. Glutamine: commercially essential or conditionally essential? A critical appraisal of the human data. *Am Jour Clin Nutr.* 2001;74:25-32.
4. De-Souza D, Greene,L. Pharmacological Nutrition After Burn Injury. *Jour Nutr.* 1998;128:797-803.
5. D'Souza, R, Powell-Tuck, J. Glutamine supplements in the critically ill. *J Royal Soc Med.* 2004; 97:425-427.
6. Frank S, Kampfer H, Wetzler C, Pfeilschifter J. Nitric oxide drives skin repair: Novel functions of an established mediator. *Kidney International.* 2002;61:882-888.
7. Miller, A. Therapeutic Considerations of L-Glutamine: A Review of the Literature. *Alternative Medicine Review.* 1999;4:239-248.
8. Morris, S. Arginine: beyond protein. *Amer J Clin Nutr.* 2006;83(suppl):508S-512S.
9. Newsholme, P. Why is L-Glutamine Metabolism Important to Cells of the Immune System in Health, Postinjury, Surgery or Infection. *Jour Nutr.* 2001;131:2515S-2522S.
10. Stechmiller J, Childress B, Porter T. Arginine Immunonutrition in Critically Ill Patients: A Clinical Dilemma. *Am Jour Crit Care.* 2004;13:17-23.
11. Wilmore, D. Enteral and Parenteral Arginine Supplementation to Improve Medical Outcomes in Hospitalized Patients. *Jour Nutr.* 2004;134: 2863S-2867S.
12. Wilmore, D. The Effect of Glutamine Supplementation in Patients Following Elective Surgery and Accidental Injury. *Jour Nutr.* 2001;131:2543S-2549S.
13. Schulman AS, Willcutts KF, Claridge JA, Evans HL, Radigan AE, O'Donnell KB, Camden JR, Chong TW, McElearney ST, Smith RL, Gazoni LM, Farinholt HM, Heuser CC, Lowson SM, Schirmer BD, Young JS, Sawyer RG. Does the addition of glutamine to enteral feeds affect patient mortality? *Crit Care Med.* 2005;33(11):2501-2506.
14. Marik PE, Zaloga GP. Immunonutrition in critically ill patients: a systematic review and analysis of the literature. *Intensive Care Med.* 2008;34(11):1980-1990.
15. Metheney NM. Twenty ways to prevent tube feeding complications. *Nurs.* 1985;47-50.
16. McClave SA, Snider HL, Lowen CC, *et al.* Use of residual volume as a marker for enteral feed tolerance: Prospective blinded comparison with physical examination and radiographic findings. *J Parenter Enteral Nutr.* 1992;16:99-105.

17. Brotherton AM, Judd PA. Quality of life in adult enteral tube feeding patients. *J Hum Nutr Diet.* 2007;20(6):513-522.
18. Brotherton A, Abbott J, Aggett P. The impact of percutaneous endoscopic gastrostomy feeding upon daily life in adults. *J Hum Nutr Diet.* 2006;19(5):355-367.
19. Williams NT. Medication administration through enteral feeding tubes. *Am J Health Syst Pharm.* 2008;65(24):2347-2357.
20. Phillips NM, Nay R. A systematic review of nursing administration of medication via enteral tubes in adults. *J Clin Nurs.* 2008;17(17):2257-2265.
21. Magnuson BL, Clifford TM, Hoskins LA, Bernard AC. Enteral nutrition and drug administration, interactions, and complications. *Nutr Clin Pract.* 2005;20(6):618-624.
22. Hennessy DD. Recovery of phenytoin from feeding formulas and protein mixtures. *Am J Health Syst Pharm.* 2003;60(18):1850-1852.
23. Burstein AH, Cox DS, Mistry B, Eddington ND. Phenytoin pharmacokinetics following oral administration of phenytoin suspension and fosphenytoin solution to rats. *Epilepsy Res.* 1999;34(2-3):129-133.
24. Kitchen D, Smith D. Problems with phenytoin administration in neurology/neurosurgery ITU patients receiving enteral feeding. *Seizure.* 2001;10(4):265-268.
25. Au Yeung SC, Ensom MH. Phenytoin and enteral feedings: does evidence support an interaction? *Ann Pharmacother.* 2000;34(7-8):896-905.
26. Doak KK, Haas CE, Dunnigan KJ, Reiss RA, Reiser JR, Huntress J, Altavela JL. Bioavailability of phenytoin acid and phenytoin sodium with enteral feedings. *Pharmacotherapy.* 1998;18(3):637-645.
27. Faraji B, Yu PP. Serum phenytoin levels of patients on gastrostomy tube feeding. *J Neurosci Nurs.* 1998;30(1):55-59.
28. Bankhead, R., Boullata, J., Brantley, S., Corkins, M., Guenter, P., Krenitsky, J., & Wessel, J. ASPEN Enteral Nutrition Practice Recommendations. JPEN Journal Of Parenteral & Enteral Nutrition. March 2009; 33(2):122-167.
29. Deane AM, Fraser RJ, Chapman MJ. Prokinetic drugs for feed intolerance in critical illness: current and potential therapies. *Crit Care Resusc.* 2009;11(2):132-143.
30. Röhm KD, Boldt J, Piper SN. Motility disorders in the ICU: recent therapeutic options and clinical practice. *Curr Opin Clin Nutr Metab Care.* 2009;12(2):161-167.
31. Landzinski J, Kiser TH, Fish DN, Wischmeyer PE, MacLaren R. Gastric motility function in critically ill patients tolerant vs intolerant to gastric nutrition. *JPEN J Parenter Enteral Nutr.* 2008;32(1):45-50.
32. Deane A, Young R. Comment on: The use of erythromycin as a gastrointestinal prokinetic agent in adult critical care: benefits versus risks. *Antimicrob Chemother.* 2008 Jan;61(1):227.
33. Nguyen NQ, Chapman M, Fraser RJ, Bryant LK, Burgstad C, Holloway RH. Prokinetic therapy for feed intolerance in critical illness: one drug or two? *Crit Care Med.* 2007;35(11):2561-2567.
34. Vonberg RP, Kuijper EJ, Wilcox MH, Barbut F, Tüll P, Gastmeier P; European C difficile-Infection Control Group; European Centre for Disease Prevention and Control (ECDC), van den Broek PJ, Colville A, Coignard B, Daha T, Debast S, Duerden BI, van den Hof S, van der Kooi T, Maarleveld HJ, Nagy E, Notermans DW, O'Driscoll J, Patel B, Stone S, Wiuff C.

Infection control measures to limit the spread of Clostridium difficile. _Clin Microbiol Infect._ 2008;14 Suppl 5:2-20.

35. Taslim H. Clostridium difficile infection in the elderly. _Acta Med Indones._ 2009;41(3):148-51.

36. Bauer MP, van Dissel JT, Kuijper EJ. Clostridium difficile: controversies and approaches to management. _Curr Opin Infect Dis._ 2009 Sep 4.

37. Rushdi TA, Pichard C, Khater YH. Control of diarrhea by fiber-enriched diet in ICU patients on enteral nutrition: a prospective randomized controlled trial. _Clin Nutr._ 2004;23(6):1344-1352.

38. Elia M, Engfer MB, Green CJ, Silk DB. Systematic review and meta-analysis: the clinical and physiological effects of fibre-containing enteral formulae. _Aliment Pharmacol Ther._ 2008;27(2):120-415.

39. Mateo MA. Nursing management of enteral tube feedings. _Heart Lung._ 1996;25(4):318-323.

40. Bommarito A, Boysen D, Heinzelman M. Unclogging feeding tubes with pancreatic enzyme. _JPEN J Parenter Enteral Nutr._ 1990;14(6):668-669.

41. Marcuard SP, Stegall KS. Unclogging feeding tubes with pancreatic enzyme. _JPEN J Parenter Enteral Nutr._ 1990;14(2):198-200.

42. Metheny N, Eisenberg P, McSweeney M. Effect of feeding tube properties and three irrigants on clogging rates. _Nurs Res._ 1988;37(3):165-169.

43. Nicholson LJ. Declogging small-bore feeding tubes. _JPEN J Parenter Enteral Nutr._ 1987;11(6):594-597.

44. McClave SA, Lukan JK, Stefater JA, Lowen CC, Looney SW, Matheson PJ, Gleeson K, Spain DA. Poor validity of residual volumes as a marker for risk of aspiration in critically ill patients. _Crit Care Med._ 2005;33(2):324-330.

45. Gaur S, Sorg T, Shukla V. Systemic absorption of FD&C blue dye associated with patient mortality. _Postgrad Med J._ 2003;79(936):602-603.

46. Lucarelli MR, Shirk MB, Julian MW, Crouser ED. Toxicity of Food Drug and Cosmetic Blue No. 1 dye in critically ill patients. _Chest._ 2004;125(2):793-795.

47. Klein L. Is blue dye safe as a method of detection for pulmonary aspiration? _J Am Diet Assoc._ 2004;104(11):1651-1652.

48. Blei AT. Diagnosis and treatment of hepatic encephalopathy. _Baillieres Best Pract Res Clin Gastroenterol._ 2000;14(6):959-74.

49. Blei AT, Cordoba J. Hepatic Encephalopathy. _Am J Gastroenterol._ 2001;96(7):1968-76. Charlton M. Branched-chain amino acid enriched supplements as therapy for liver disease. _J Nutr._ 2006;136(1 Suppl):295S-8S.

50. Chatauret N, ButterworthRF. Effects of liver failure on inter-organ trafficking of ammonia: implications for the treatment of hepatic encephalopathy. _J Gastroenterol Hepatol._ 2004;19:219-223.

51. Cordoba J, Lopez-Hellin J, Planas M, Sabin P, Sanpedro F, Castro F, et al. Normal protein diet for episodic hepatic encephalopathy: results of a randomized study. _J Hepatol._ 2004;41(1):38-43.

52. Dejong CH, van de Poll MC, Soeters PB, Jalan R, Olde Damink SW. Aromatic amino acid metabolism during liver failure. _J Nutr._ 2007;137(6 Suppl 1):1579S-85S; discussion 97S-98S.

53. Ferenci P, Lockwood A, Mullen K, Tarter R, Weissenborn K, Blei AT. Hepatic encephalopathy--definition, nomenclature, diagnosis, and quantification: final report of the working party at the 11th World Congresses of Gastroenterology, Vienna, 1998. *Hepatology.* 2002;35(3):716-21.
54. Malaguarnera M, Pistone G, Elvira R, Leotta C, Scarpello L, Liborio R. Effects of L-carnitine in patients with hepatic encephalopathy. *World J Gastroenterol.* 2005;11(45):7197-202.
55. Marchesini G, Bianchi G, Merli M, Amodio P, Panella C, Loguercio C, et al. Nutritional supplementation with branched-chain amino acids in advanced cirrhosis: a double-blind, randomized trial. *Gastroenterology.* 2003;124(7):1792-801.
56. Marchesini G, Fabbri A, Bianchi G, Brizi M, Zoli M. Zinc supplementation and amino acid-nitrogen metabolism in patients with advanced cirrhosis. *Hepatology.* 1996;23(5):1084-92.
57. Marchesini G, Marzocchi R, Noia M, Bianchi G. Branched-chain amino acid supplementation in patients with liver diseases. *J Nutr.* 2005;135(6 Suppl):1596S-601S.
58. Mizock, BA. Nutritional support in hepatic encephalopathy. *Nutrition.* 1999;15(3): 220-8.
59. Nakaya Y, Okita K, Suzuki K, Moriwaki H, Kato A, Miwa Y, et al. BCAA-enriched snack improves nutritional state of cirrhosis. *Nutrition.* 2007;23(2):113-20.
60. O'Brien A, Williams R. Nutrition in end-stage liver disease: principles and practice. *Gastroenterology.* 2008;134(6):1729-40.
61. Prasad S, Dhiman RK, Duseja A, Chawla YK, Sharma A, Agarwal R. Lactulose improves cognitive functions and health-related quality of life in patients with cirrhosis who have minimal hepatic encephalopathy. *Hepatology.* 2007;45(3):549-59.
62. Tsiaousi ET, Hatzitolios AI, Trygonis SK, Savopoulos CG. Malnutrition in end stage liver disease: recommendations and nutritional support. *J Gastroenterol Hepatol.* 2008;23(4):527-33.
63. Watanabe A, Sakai T, Sato S, Imai F, Ohto M, Arakawa Y, et al. Clinical efficacy of lactulose in cirrhotic patients with and without subclinical hepatic encephalopathy. *Hepatology.* 1997;26(6):1410-4.
64. Yang SS, Lai YC, Chiang TR, Chen DF, Chen DS. Role of zinc in subclinical hepatic encephalopathy: comparison with somatosensory-evoked potentials. *J Gastroenterol Hepatol.* 2004;19(4):375-9.
65. Plauth M, Cabré E, Campillo B, Kondrup J, Marchesini G, Schütz T, Shenkin A, Wendon J. ESPEN Guidelines on Parenteral Nutrition: hepatology. *Clin Nutr.* 2009;28(4):436-444.
66. American Society for Parenteral and Enteral Nutrition. Clinical Guidelines. Retrieved 06 August 2015. http://www.nutritioncare.org/

Children with Special Health Care Needs

1. Krebs NF, Himes JH, Jacobson D, Nicklas TA, Guilday P, Styne D. Assessment of child and adolescent overweight and obesity. *Pediatrics.* 2007;120 Suppl 4:S193-228.
2. Mintzer S, Skidmore CT, Abidin CJ, Morales MC, Chervoneva I, Capuzzi DM, Sperling MR. Effects of antiepileptic drugs on lipids, homocysteine, and C-reactive protein. *Ann Neurol.* 2009;65(4):448-456.
3. Sener U, Zorlu Y, Karaguzel O, Ozdamar O, Coker I, Topbas M. Effects of common anti-epileptic drug monotherapy on serum levels of homocysteine, vitamin B12, folic acid and vitamin B6. *Seizure.* 2006;15(2):79-85.

4. Faraone SV, Biederman J, Morley CP, Spencer TJ. Effect of stimulants on height and weight: a review of the literature. *J Am Acad Child Adolesc Psychiatry.* 2008;47(9):994-1009.

5. Poulton A, Cowell CT. Slowing of growth in height and weight on stimulants: a characteristic pattern. *J Paediatr Child Health.* 2003;39(3):180-185.

6. Loening-Baucke V. Functional constipation. *Seminars in Pediatric Surgery.* 1995;4: 26-34.

7. Loening-Baucke V. Constipation in children. *Curr Opin Pediatr.* 1994;6(5):556-561.

8. Loening-Baucke V, Swidsinski A. Constipation as cause of acute abdominal pain in children. *J Pediatr.* 2007;151(6):666-669.

9. Mosby TT, Barr RD, Pencharz PB. Nutritional assessment of children with cancer. *J Pediatr Oncol Nurs.* 2009;26(4):186-97.

10. Sala A, Pencharz P, Barr RD. Children, cancer, and nutrition--A dynamic triangle in review. *Cancer.* 2004;100(4):677-687.

11. Edefonti A, Mastrangelo A, Paglialonga F. Assessment and monitoring of nutrition status in pediatric peritoneal dialysis patients. *Perit Dial Int.* 2009;29 Suppl 2:S176-9.

12. Srivaths PR, Wong C, Goldstein SL. Nutrition aspects in children receiving maintenance hemodialysis: impact on outcome. *Pediatr Nephrol.* 2009 May;24(5):951-957.

13. Terrill CJ. Nutrition and the pediatric patient with CKD. *Nephrol Nurs J.* 2007 Jan-Feb;34(1):89-92.

14. Rees L, Shaw V. Nutrition in children with CRF and on dialysis. *Pediatr Nephrol.* 2007;22(10):1689-1702.

15. Miller D, MacDonald D. Management of pediatric patients with chronic kidney disease. *Pediatr Nurs.* 2006;32(2):128-34; quiz 135.

16. Gisel E. Interventions and outcomes for children with dysphagia. *Dev Disabil Res Rev.* 2008;14(2):165-73.

17. Kuperminc MN, Stevenson RD. Growth and nutrition disorders in children with cerebral palsy. *Dev Disabil Res Rev.* 2008;14(2):137-146.

18. Hogan SE. Energy requirements of children with cerebral palsy. *Can J Diet Pract Res.* 2004;65(3):124-30.

19. Rogers B. Feeding method and health outcomes of children with cerebral palsy. *J Pediatr.* 2004;145(2 Suppl):S28-32.

20. Truby H, Cowlishaw P, O'Neil C, Wainwright C. The long term efficacy of gastrostomy feeding in children with cystic fibrosis on anthropometric markers of nutritonal status and pulmonary function. *Open Respir Med J.* 2009;3:112-115.

21. Nasr SZ, Drury D. Appetite stimulants use in cystic fibrosis. *Pediatr Pulmonol.* 2008;43(3):209-219.

22. Kalnins D, Durie PR, Pencharz P. Nutritional management of cystic fibrosis patients. *Curr Opin Clin Nutr Metab Care.* 2007;10(3):348-354.

23. Lai HJ. Classification of nutritional status in cystic fibrosis. *Curr Opin Pulm Med.* 2006;12(6):422-7.

24. Davidson ZE, Truby H. A review of nutrition in Duchenne muscular dystrophy. *J Hum Nutr Diet.* 2009;22(5):383-393.

25. Miller CK. Updates on pediatric feeding and swallowing problems. *Curr Opin Otolaryngol Head Neck Surg.* 2009;17(3):194-199.

26. Arvedson JC. Assessment of pediatric dysphagia and feeding disorders: clinical and instrumental approaches. *Dev Disabil Res Rev.* 2008;14(2):118-127.
27. Cooper-Brown L, Copeland S, Dailey S, Downey D, Petersen MC, Stimson C, Van Dyke DC. Feeding and swallowing dysfunction in genetic syndromes. *Dev Disabil Res Rev.* 2008;14(2):147-157.
28. Hartman C, Eliakim R, Shamir R. Nutritional status and nutritional therapy in inflammatory bowel diseases. *World J Gastroenterol.* 2009;15(21):2570-2578.
29. El-Matary W. Enteral nutrition as a primary therapy of Crohn's disease: the pediatric perspective. *Nutr Clin Pract.* 2009;24(1):91-97.
30. Walia R, Mahajan L, Steffen R. Recent advances in chronic constipation. *Curr Opin Pediatr.* 2009 Jul 13.

Adverse Reactions to Food

1. Food Allergy Research and Education. About Food Allergies. Retrieved 06 August 2015. http://www.foodallergy.org/about-food-allergies.
2. Ramesh S. Food allergy overview in children. *Clin Rev Allergy Immunol.* 2008;34:217-230 .
3. Food Allergen Labeling and Consumer Protection Act of 2004 (Title II of Public Law 108-282) http://www.cfsan.fda.gov/~dms/alrgact.html Accessed April 10, 2009.

Louisiana Academy of Nutrition and Dietetics
Manual of Medical Nutrition Therapy

Policies

The Diet Manual Committee wishes to make clear that (1) any member of the Louisiana Academy of Nutrition and Dietetics (LAND) may copy (observing all applicable guidelines) the information in the *LAND Manual of Medical Nutrition Therapy* for educational and instructional purposes without obtaining permission from the editor to do so, and (2) the format and any written material in the *LAND Manual of Medical Nutrition Therapy* is copyrighted and subject to the guidelines below.

1. Non-LAND members and other associations and organizations wishing to copy portions of the 2010 edition of the *LAND Manual of Medical Nutrition* Therapy must request permission in writing from:

    Editor
    LAND Manual of Medical Nutrition Therapy
    The Louisiana Dietetic Association
    8550 United Plaza Boulevard, Suite 1001
    Baton Rouge, LA 70809

The request should state what page or pages are to be copied and the reason or need to copy, *e.g.* classes for dietetic interns. The editor will act on each request.

1. After receiving the written request, basic policy will be to grant permission to copy pages or sections of the manual that will be used for patient instructions, classes for medical students, dietetic interns or students or for other educational reasons (intent must be specified).
2. Other dietetic associations or non-profit organizations that request permission to incorporate part of the Manual in diet manuals they are compiling will be handled on an individual basis. Sections and/or pages must be specified in the request. Basic policy will be to grant permission to other dietetic associations to use copyrighted material in their manuals without charge as long as credit is given to the Louisiana Dietetic Association.
3. Requests to copy received from profit making organizations such as drug companies or publishing companies will be handled on an individual basis. Basic policy will be to levy a per page charge. Requests should be sent to the Editor at the above address.
4. If the use of copyrighted materials is done verbatim, the page should carry the copyrighted line as it appears in the Manual. If it is an adaptation, the line should read: "Adapted with permission from the *LAND Manual of Medical Nutrition Therapy*, 2015 Edition."

Permission to Copy

Guidelines for copying are stated in the LAND Manual of Medical Nutrition Therapy. Send this completed form to:

Editor
LAND Manual of Medical Nutrition Therapy
The Louisiana Academy of Nutrition and Dietetics
8550 United Plaza Boulevard, Suite 1001
Baton Rouge, LA 70809

Name_____

Organization _____

Profit or Non-profit (Circle one)

Pages to Copy _____

Intended Use of Copied Material: _____

Signature _____ Date _____

2 GRAM Sodium Diet (2000 mg)

Your doctor has recommended that you follow a 2 gram sodium diet. This will help your body to eliminate any excess water that it may be retaining. This diet is often used in cases of high blood pressure, congestive heart failure, kidney disease, or liver disease.

GENERAL DESCRIPTION

A low sodium diet restricts foods prepared or served with salt. Foods that contain high amounts of sodium are omitted.

RECOMMENDATIONS

1. Do not add salt to foods during cooking or at the table.

2. Only use a salt substitute if your doctor says it is okay.

3. Avoid instant or quick-cook foods. These types of foods are generally high in sodium.

4. Avoid canned or instant soups, stews, chili, and bouillon cubes, unless products are labeled as low sodium.

Patient's Name _____   Date _____

RD _____   Phone _____

CARDIAC DIET

Your doctor has recommended that you follow a cardiac diet. This diet is used in the management of chronic heart disease.

GUIDELINES

1. Achieve and maintain a desirable body weight.
2. Decrease the amount of fat in your diet, especially saturated fat. Saturated fat is found in animal products, whole milk dairy products, and some oils.
3. Choose lean cuts of meat with the fat trimmed (skinless chicken and turkey, fish).
4. Use skim or 1% milk, and cheeses with no more than 2 to 6 grams of fat per ounce.
5. Limit egg yolks to 3 per week.
6. Avoid using butter, lard, bacon fat, coconut, and palm kernel oils. Instead, use corn, olive, peanut, canola, safflower, sesame, and soybean oils. Use tub (not stick) margarine. Limit intake of nuts, seeds, avocados, and olives.
7. Most breads, bagels, English muffins, low fat crackers, cereals, noodles, rice, beans, and peas are low in fat. However, avoid adding fats to these foods. Croissants, sweet rolls, pastries, crackers made with saturated oils, granola cereals, and egg noodles are higher in fat and should not be eaten.
8. Fruits and vegetables are a good choice for a snack or as part of a meal. Avoid vegetables prepared in butter, cream, or sauces which are high in fat.
9. Avoid eating too many sweets. For dessert, choose low fat options such as sherbet, sorbet, frozen yogurt, angel food cake, gingersnaps, plain popcorn, pretzels, low fat jelly beans, and hard candy.

Patient's Name _____   Date _____

RD _____   Phone _____

DIABETIC DIET

Your doctor has recommended that you follow a diabetic diet to help control your blood sugar levels. This diet may also aid in weight reduction and improving your blood lipid levels.

GUIDELINES

1. Achieve and maintain an ideal body weight. This will help you better control your diabetes.
2. Avoid eating concentrated sweets, such as sugar, honey, jelly, candy, dried fruit, and sweetened cereals. Concentrated sweets will cause your blood sugar level to rise quickly.
3. Limit the use of "dietetic" cookies, candy, or cakes to 1 to 2 servings per day or about 60 calories per day. These foods maybe high in fat and calories and include other sweeteners.
4. Do not skip or delay meals. Eat regularly scheduled meals.
5. Eat more complex carbohydrates such as bread, pasta, rice, potatoes, and beans.
6. Include plenty of fiber in your diet. Whole grain breads and cereals, fruits and vegetables will provide fiber.
7. Reduce your intake of saturated fat and cholesterol. Foods high in saturated fat and cholesterol include fatty meats, liver, butter, lard, bacon grease, and fat back.
8. Avoid drinking alcohol or beer.

Patient's Name _____   Date _____

RD _____   Phone _____

204

INCREASING CALORIES IN YOUR DIET

Your doctor has recommended that you increase calories and protein in your diet. It is important that you maintain good nutritional status so that you can be stronger, your body can fight infections, and you can feel better.

RECOMMENDATIONS

1. Eat three meals a day with snacks.
2. Use commercial supplements, such as Ensure or Boost, to provide additional calories, protein, and other nutrients. Ask your doctor or dietitian which one is right for you.
3. Add dry skim milk powder to casseroles and other recipes when cooking.
4. Use whipped topping to garnish desserts.
5. Add grated cheese to grits, vegetables, and starchy foods.
6. Add margarine and gravy to foods.
7. Eat double portions of foods that you like, such as desserts.
8. Use Half & Half to make puddings.
9. Prepare Jell-O with fruit or applesauce.
10. Cook dry cereals with milk instead of water.

Patient's Name _____   Date _____

RD _____   Phone _____

Made in the USA
San Bernardino, CA
24 May 2016